ADDICTION

ADDICTION

A Disorder of Choice

GENE M. HEYMAN

HARVARD UNIVERSITY PRESS

Cambridge, Massachusetts, and London, England

First Harvard University Press paperback edition, 2010

Library of Congress Cataloging-in-Publication Data

Heyman, Gene M.
Addiction : a disorder of choice / Gene M. Heyman.
p.   cm.
Includes bibliographical references and index.
ISBN 978-0-674-03298-9 (cloth : alk. paper)
ISBN 978-0-674-05727-2 (pbk.)
1. Drug addiction.   2. Compulsive behavior.   I. Title.
HV5801.H459   2009
616.86001—dc22   2009003752

CONTENTS

PREFACE

This is a book about addiction. It is also a book about those behaviors that we choose to do—which restaurant to go to, what subject to major in, whom to marry—that is, it is also a book about voluntary behavior. Addiction also helps us understand voluntary behavior; it shines a light on its dark sides. The two go together, I propose, because it is not possible to understand addiction without understanding how we make choices. To be sure, it is unlikely that anyone chooses to be an addict, but what research shows is that everyone, including those who are called addicts, stops using drugs when the costs of continuing become too great. This paradox is at the heart of the understanding of choice and also at the heart of understanding addiction. In everyday speech this paradox is avoided. According to the dictionary, "addiction" is compulsive drug use, and by definition, "compulsive" acts are "irresistible" acts. In contrast, voluntary acts are resistible; you don't have to eat out at a restaurant tonight, you can major in English rather than in engineering, and so on. On the basis of conversations and formal presentations at research meetings, most addiction experts agree with the everyday understanding of addiction. In technical research papers and clinical texts, addiction is referred to as a "chronic, relapsing brain disease." What the public and professionals say about addiction is important. Federal agencies have spent billions of taxpayer dollars on addiction, and thousands of trained professionals have dedicated their careers to solving the "drug problem." If addiction has not been properly defined, then it is likely that these efforts are not accomplishing as much as they could. It may be that addicts are affected by what appears in the research and clinical journals. It probably makes a difference whether someone seeking help for a drug problem is told that he or she has a chronic, relapsing brain disease, or that most heavy drug users manage to quit, and with help it is possible to quit sooner rather than later.

I have arranged the material in this book so that the readers can determine the nature of addiction for themselves. One chapter presents the natural history of addiction, using the words of addicts to tell the story. Other chapters introduce research findings that are most relevant to understanding the natural history of addiction, such as the likelihood that addicts quit using drugs and the circumstances under which this occurs. The research results are summarized in graphs. In many cases, it is possible to compare the results from different studies to see if the findings are reliable. For topics in which different researchers used different methods, it is possible to test if the findings reflect the methods or the nature of drug use itself. For example, on the basis of national epidemiological survey results, it is possible to check whether the themes that emerged in the autobiographies of addicts reflect typical life histories or the idiosyncratic tales of a small group of drug addicts who like to talk to researchers.

This book's approach to voluntary behavior is more conceptual than its approach to addiction. It begins with three general principles and then uses them to derive basic properties of voluntary behavior. As in the discussion of addiction, one of my reasons for taking this approach is transparency. The reader can judge whether the initial assumptions are, as claimed, "self-evident" and "general," and likewise the reader can evaluate the manner in which the principles were combined to generate the predictions. The most important prediction is that "on paper" the rules of voluntary behavior yield patterns of drug taking that correspond to clinical accounts of addiction. For example, the analysis says that we should expect periods of heavy drug use to alternate with periods of abstinence. This agrees with clinical reports.

The book also includes an introduction to the history of opiate use and ideas about addiction. The historical material is arranged to answer the following questions: How long have opiates been used? When did addiction first appear on a national scale? When did the idea that addiction is a disease first emerge? What is the basis for the idea that drug use can become involuntary? As we will see, how people have thought about what a disease is and whether getting drunk or high could be symptomatic of a disease state were themselves symptomatic of more general understandings regarding the nature of choice and individual responsibility.

Most of the research that I review in this book concerns illegal drugs, primarily opiates and stimulants. Legal drugs are discussed, but usually they are not the focus. The distinction is consistent with the main research findings. A drug's legal status influences choices concerning its use, so that the story of alcohol and cigarette use differs significantly from the story of opiate and stimulant use. Consequently, to have given legal drugs as much weight as illegal ones would have required a much longer book. However, the basic ideas presented here apply to alcohol and cigarettes, and there are instances in which aspects of alcohol and cigarette use are most relevant to the issues under discussion. For instance, the section on what makes a substance addictive includes an extended discussion of why cigarettes are considered addictive even though they are not intoxicating.

Many individuals helped complete this book. First and foremost, I am happy to have this opportunity to thank my wife, Martha Pott, for her patient, careful, and wise advice on each of the chapters, in each of their many versions. I would also like to thank Phoebe Pott-Heyman for her editorial help and detective work tracking down errant citations. I am indebted to Verna Mims, who established the core reference list and has been invaluable in helping with the book and the courses that I teach related to this book. Thanks to Jerry Zuriff, my friend and colleague, for his critical comments and good humor. A number of colleagues and friends provided careful readings and helpful comments on the individual chapters: Brian Dunn, Samantha Gibb, Paul Harris, Jim Hopper, Jim Mazur, Hal Miller, and Steve Negus. Their effort and time are greatly appreciated. Conversations with Tony Volpe and Pirooz Vakili were fun and stimulating and contributed to the quantitative analyses that guide Chapters 6 and 7. Many thanks to my editor, Elizabeth Knoll. She was instrumental in steering the book into its present form and kept the project going in face of serious challenges. Also many thanks to Kate Brick, the manuscript editor. She scrupulously and wisely copyedited the manuscript, markedly improving the text. I am indebted to Patrick Griswold and the staff at the North Charles Institute for the Addictions Narcotics Treatment Program for their hospitality and instruction. Eric Wanner and the Russell Sage Foundation generously supported the project at its onset. I remain appreciative and indebted to their contribution. It also should be said that this book would not have been written had it not been for Richard Herrnstein's pioneering research on choice and the support and encouragement he generously offered me and several generations of graduate students who began their research careers in his laboratory.

ADDICTION

1

RESPONSES TO ADDICTION

In 1914 the United States Congress passed a law that authorized the federal government to regulate the distribution of opiates and cocaine. Since then official U.S. policy regarding addictive drugs and addiction has involved both the judicial system and the country's health institutes. The judicial system prosecutes drug users and drug dealers, often sending them to jail; the medical system treats drug users, sending them to clinics and hospitals. Each strategy has a powerful institutional presence. The Drug Enforcement Agency is a multibillion-dollar-per-year bureaucracy in the Department of Justice. The National Institute on Drug Abuse is a billion-dollar-per-year research and service component of the National Institutes of Health (NIH). Although each agency is highly respected and well established, that two such different bureaucracies have responsibility for addictive drugs suggests that there is something amiss in the American response to addiction. We typically do not advocate incarceration and medical care for the same activities. Indeed, addiction is the only psychiatric syndrome whose symptoms—illicit drug use—are considered an illegal activity, and conversely addictive drug use is the only illegal activity that is also the focus of highly ambitious research and treatment programs.

As addiction emerged as a specialized area of study and treatment, experts found fault with the role of the judicial system. August Vollmer, one of the founders of the study of criminology and the practice of law enforcement, was an early critic of the Harrison Narcotics Tax Act of 1914, which regulated and taxed the production, importation, and distribution of opiates. In 1936 he wrote that the legal prohibitions had forced "the helpless addict . . . to resort to crime in order to get money for the drug which is absolutely indispensable for his comfortable existence . . . Drug addiction . . . is not a police problem . . . It is first and last a medical problem" (cited in Brecher, 1972, pp. 52–53). A few years later, Alfred Lindesmith, one of the first academics to specialize in the study of addiction, took a similar position: "punishment and imprisonment of addicts is as cruel and pointless as similar treatment for persons infected with syphilis . . . The treatment of addicts in the United States is on no higher plane than the persecution of witches in other ages" (cited in Brecher, 1972, p. 53). Vollmer was a policeman and Lindesmith was a sociologist, yet both believed that the justice department had no place in the response to addiction because addiction was more akin to a disease or psychiatric disorder than a crime. In fact, according to Vollmer the prohibitions are what established the connection between addiction and criminal activity. Today, the idea that addiction is a disease has become widely accepted, but curiously this has not undermined the justice department's role in addiction. The number of people in jail for drug offenses has steadily increased and is currently at an all-time high.

Criticisms of punitive jail sentences for addicts make perfect sense if the prohibitions are what established the connection between addiction and crime. However, the history of drug use in the United States reveals a more complicated story. The connection between addictive drug use and criminality was in place before federal laws banned opiate and cocaine use. Similarly, the view that addictive drug use was a disease also emerged prior to the beginning of scientific research on addictive drugs. From the start, addiction invited both legal prohibitions and the impulse to cure it. This does not mean that addiction is in fact a crime or a disease, but it raises the possibility that there is more to the current two-pronged approach to addiction than misunderstanding and the inappropriate use of punishment.

As a first step toward a reconsideration of the nature of addiction, this chapter traces key features of illicit drug use in the United States prior to the first legal prohibitions. The history reveals that the current approach made sense at the time it was first formulated. The historical sketch is then followed by an overview of the costs that addictive drugs exact on society, as measured in terms of distress and dollars. These results show why it is so important to come to a better understanding of addiction. Addictive drugs promote chaotic and unhappy social relations, result in many serious medical problems (including HIV/AIDS), and have led to social policies that are more notable for their costs than their effectiveness.

Opiate Use Prior to the Harrison Act

In the nineteenth and early twentieth centuries Americans who became ill tended to medicate themselves rather than seek out professional help. The self-treatments of choice were patent medicines, whose active ingredients included alcohol, opiates, and cocaine. These potions were unregulated and advertised as essential and healthful. Those who lived in towns and cities could go to their local pharmacy and buy these various intoxicating "medicines." Those not near a pharmacy could order the drugs by mail from Sears, Roebuck and Company and other national emporiums. The product names were colorful and innocent: Mrs. Winslow's Soothing Syrup, Dover Powder, McMunn's Elixir of Opium, Heroin Cough Sedatives, and Cocaine Toothache Drops.

One book refers to America during this period as a "dope fiend's paradise" (Brecher, 1972). The period is also a boon for historical research. It offers the opportunity to investigate longstanding questions regarding the influence of drug prohibitions on drug use and their social consequences. For instance, were addiction rates at epidemically high levels? In the absence of prohibitions, were addicts no less law-abiding than their sober peers? The period establishes what is sometimes called a "natural experiment," in this case a test of the effects of decriminalizing drugs. But we should be forewarned that a "natural experiment" is a contradiction in terms. The essence of an experiment is the capacity to control the independent variables while holding their correlates constant, which we can't do in this case. Also, in the late nineteenth and early twentieth centuries, there were no psychiatric epidemiologists collecting data on addiction, so the available information is not systematic or comprehensive.

On the basis of the sales and a few medical surveys, David Courtwright (1982), who has written the most detailed account of American drug use prior to 1914, estimates that opiate addiction peaked in the 1890s at a prevalence rate of approximately 4.6 addicts per thousand persons. The figure is surprising in two regards. First, the peak occurs well before the 1914 prohibitions went into effect, and second, the number is not so different from current estimates of opiate addiction. For example, the most recent national survey, conducted over the years 2001 and 2002, reports that there were about 3.4 opiate addicts per thousand persons and about 10.8

nonaddicted heavy opiate users (these are lifetime rates, meaning both current and ex-addicts; Conway et al., 2006).

The researchers who carried out the recent survey went to great lengths to establish a representative sample of subjects and interviewed more than 40,000 informants (National Epidemiologic Survey on Alcohol and Related Conditions [NESARC]; Grant et al., 2006), whereas Courtwright had to rely on limited, unscientific sources, such as sales and import ledgers. Possibly, then, the nineteenth-century rates were higher than the available data suggest. However, for the purpose of trying to make sense of why addiction is a matter of great concern for both the Department of Justice and the National Institutes of Health, the actual numbers are not as important as who used opiates. This is a question of demographics, and the demographic correlates of nineteenth-century opiate use are better understood than its quantitative features. According to various late-nineteenth-century sources, there were three types of opiate addicts: "opium eaters," who drank tinctures composed of opiates and alcohol; opium smokers; and heroin "sniffers," who inhaled the drug intranasally. The differences in self-administration techniques were accompanied by important demographic differences. The result is three distinct addiction syndromes. Two, as we will see, provide an inviting target for the punitive approach to addiction, and the other supports the medical approach.

Laudanum drinkers ("opium eaters"). In sixteenth-century medical texts, "laudanum" referred to mixtures of opium and alcohol. In nineteenth-century America, the term had the same meaning, although morphine, which is about ten times more potent than opium, was often substituted for opium. Laudanum attracted a wide range of users: male, female, older, younger, and the well-to-do. In the public's eye, laudanum was a refined, sophisticated indulgence. For example, a 1881 editorial in the *Catholic World* labeled laudanum drinking an "aristocratic vice" more common among the educated and wealthy, although the writer goes on to say that it spares no one:

> Opium-eating, unlike the use of alcoholic stimulants, is an aristocratic vice and prevails more extensively among the wealthy and educated classes than among those of inferior social position; but no class is exempt from its blighting influence. The

merchant, lawyer, and physician are to be found among the host who sacrifice the choicest treasures of life at the shrine of Opium. The slaves of Alcohol may be clothed in rags, but vassals of the monarch who sits enthroned on the poppy are generally found dressed in purple and fine linen. (quoted in Brecher, 1972, p. 18)

In keeping with laudanum's upper-class patina, physicians often played a role in the etiology of laudanum addiction. Morphine was the first "wonder drug," and it and laudanum were what physicians prescribed for a wide range of ailments. Consequently, a visit to the doctor often resulted in a daily regime of opiates. Some patients became addicted. A book published in 1868, titled *The Opium Habit* (Horace Day), includes a description of the typical sequence of events:

> The frequent, if not the usual history of confirmed opium-eaters is this: A physician prescribes opium as an anodyne, and the patient finds from its use the relief which was anticipated. Very frequently he finds not merely that his pain has been relieved, but that with this relief has been associated a feeling of positive, perhaps of extreme enjoyment. A recurrence of the same pain infallibly suggests a recurrence to the same remedy . . . He becomes his own doctor, prescribes the same remedy the medical man has prescribed, and charges nothing for his advice. The resort to this pleasant medication after no long time becomes habitual, and the patient finds that the remedy, whose use he had supposed was sanctioned by his physician, has become his tyrant. (p. 58)

The *Catholic World* and Horace Day's accounts of opium eating agree with each other and with other reports of the day (e.g., Brecher, 1972; Courtwright, 1982). However, these reports leave out a fact that is critical to understanding later developments. In contrast to opium smokers and heroin sniffers, opium eaters did not congregate among themselves. They got high in private and tried to keep their habit secret. This is important because it means that laudanum drinkers were not perceived as a threat to public safety or even a nuisance. Of course, their family and friends knew about their dependence on opiates, and because the drugs were first obtained from their physicians, their physicians probably knew as well. But this knowledge did not lead to a public outcry and call for anti-drug legislation. According to friends, relatives, and doctors, laudanum drinkers needed help, not punishment.

Opium smokers. In the mid-nineteenth century tens of thousands of Chinese immigrated to the United States to work, primarily as laborers on the transcontinental railroad and in West Coast gold and silver mines. They were poor, male, away from their families, and shunned by their new American neighbors. Opium smoking, which at the time was a serious problem in China, flourished in the mining camps, makeshift towns, and cities that became home to the Asian immigrants. In contrast to laudanum drinking, it took place with others and in public—albeit out-of-the-way—establishments referred to as "opium dens." A few non-Chinese Americans joined in. Opium smokers were considered social outsiders, not mainstream Americans as measured by ethnicity or lifestyle.

The demographic profile of the opium smokers differed markedly from laudanum drinkers. They were not fallen aristocrats. Rather, newspaper articles of the day described white male opium smokers as "evil" men and gamblers, and white female opium smokers as "ill-famed" women, that is, prostitutes (e.g., Courtwright, 1982). The Chinese were represented as menacing and came to be known as the "yellow peril." The movie *McCabe and Mrs. Miller* (1971), directed by Robert Altman, offers a vivid account of the newspaper version of nineteenth-century West Coast opium smoking. Mrs. Miller (Julie Christie) is a hard-edged, calculating proprietress of a house of ill repute; McCabe (Warren Beatty) is an itinerant gambler. They find common ground in their unconventional professions, good looks, and opium smoking—at least for a while.

Heroin sniffers. Bayer, the pharmaceutical company that developed aspirin, derived heroin from morphine and brought it to the market in 1898. The two drugs bind to the same brain receptors, but heroin is more potent, because it gets to the brain much faster. Bayer's interest in heroin was that it was a highly effective cough suppressant. This met an important need: two of the deadliest diseases at the turn of the twentieth century, pneumonia and tuberculosis, were accompanied by extended spells of coughing that were often life-threatening. Bayer had little or no concern about addiction because the employees who had tested the product did not become addicted to it. Indeed, heroin was also marketed as a "cure" for morphine addiction.

The first generation of recreational heroin users were young men who hung out in the streets of Philadelphia, Boston, New York, and other major East Coast cities. In an article published in the *New Republic* in 1916, Dr. Pearce Bailey described heroin sniffers as underemployed young men who had quit school early and often had a history of delinquency. They were, Bailey observed, committed to immediate pleasures, not careers. They liked to go to vaudeville shows, and they liked to sniff heroin. Bailey's tone suggests that the "heroin boys" were aimless and delinquent, but not serious criminal threats. For these young men, heroin functioned as a badge of identity, signifying rebelliousness and a disdain for the bland security of a humdrum, low-paying job. At the end of his article, Bailey proposed a treatment program based on relocating the "heroin boys" to a rural setting and allowing the restorative powers of agricultural work to do their magic.

Physicians and the Justice Department Push Back

The nineteenth- and early twentieth-century reactions to opiate use varied as a function of the mode of self-administration and the demographic profile of the users. The reactions were much like those today, even though the drugs were then legal.

Physicians seek a cure for inebriation. In the late eighteenth century, a number of physicians in the United States and England began calling self-destructive drug use a disease. In the United States, this movement was initiated by Benjamin Rush, a signer of the Constitution and advisor to Thomas Jefferson, who, unlike most of his medical peers, had an interest in behavioral disorders, particularly alcoholism. He believed that alcohol became a necessity as a function of drinking itself, thereby turning a voluntary drinker into an involuntary one. "[W]hen strongly urged, by one of his friends, to leave off drinking [an habitual drunkard] said, 'Were a keg of rum in one corner of a room, and were a cannon constantly discharging balls between me and it, I could not refrain from passing before that cannon, in order to get at the rum.'" (Quoted in Levine, 1978, p. 152.) Rush's perspective won few adherents in the late eighteenth century, but by the late nineteenth century, there was a critical mass of physicians who specialized in alcohol and opiate use. They labeled self-destructive drug use a disease, established a new medical journal, *Inebriety*, and formed a new medical organization, The Society for the Study and Cure of Inebriety. The founder of the British branch of the new organization, Dr. Norman Kerr, stated their position on addiction: Inebriety is "for the most part the issue of certain physical conditions . . . the natural product of a depraved, debilitated, or defective nervous organisation . . . as unmistakably a disease as is gout, or epilepsy, or insanity" (cited in Berridge, 1990, p. 106).

These ideas were not widely embraced outside of the circle of physicians who were specializing in problem drug use. According to Harry G. Levine, an historian of the modern concept of addiction (1978), the public believed that "inebriates" got drunk or high because they wanted to, not because they had to. That is, the public did not see heavy drinkers and morphine habitués as compulsive but as preferring intoxication to sobriety. In defense of the physicians, their views reflected their experience. Those who came to their offices for drug problems wanted help. Since people who seek out doctors for help are usually sick, it was reasonable to say that "inebriates" were sick as well. There was no other available label. The "inebriates" had broken no laws, were often well educated and wealthy, were not psychotic, and other than drug use, were respectable citizens. Given the available categories, "sick" seems the right one. An observation by Virginia Berridge (1990), an historian of addiction, nicely summarizes the medical response to opiate use prior to the Harrison Act. She points out that by the end of the nineteenth century, "morphine disease" was an expanding area of medical expertise and no "textbook of medicine was complete without its section on the 'morphia habit.'"

Congress takes control of opiates and cocaine. In contrast to opium eating, opium smoking and heroin sniffing attracted an unsavory crowd of gamblers, prostitutes, delinquents, and the unemployed. These demographics were associated with law enforcement, not medicine. Moreover, opium smokers and heroin sniffers did not seek out medical help. Consequently, a division emerged. Physicians attended opium eaters; law enforcement officials dealt with opium smokers and heroin sniffers, although not because of their drug use. These distinctions were institutionalized in the Harrison Act of 1914.[1]

The Harrison Narcotics Tax Act of 1914 limited the use of opiates and other addictive drugs to medical purposes only. Nothing was said about addiction, and medical purpose was not defined but identified as "professional practice."[2] Some physicians continued to prescribe opiates to long-term opiate users on the grounds that this was a proper medical treatment for addiction (Musto, 1973). Their patients, the physicians claimed, had a disease. Justice Department officials took the physicians to court. At first judges and juries in the United States sided with the physicians. But in time, the courts determined that treating addiction did not fall within the realm of "professional practice."

Although the Harrison Act did not explicitly address recreational drug use or addiction, it was enforced as if its intent was to suppress drug use and addiction. The legislative branch of government rejected the views of the Society for the Study and Cure of Inebriety. They decreed that opiate and cocaine use were not symptoms of a disease but criminal offenses. As a result, American drug use patterns were transformed. Laudanum drinkers and opium smokers all but disappeared. Heroin use persisted, but because it was now illegal, it became even more closely tied to criminal activity. Criminal gangs took over heroin's distribution, raised prices, and adulterated it with inert substances. To get the same kick that snorting heroin had provided, users now had to inject heroin. Apparently, few laudanum drinkers were willing to inject themselves with a substance that by weight was about a hundred times more powerful than opium. There were some heroin addicts who had no association with criminal activity other than heroin use itself, but they were largely invisible (see Frieda's story in Chapter 3; Courtwright et al., 1989). Street addicts were no longer "heroin boys" with a penchant for vaudeville and petty crimes, they were serious criminals. Among the first to document the transformation of opiate use in America were Lawrence Kolb and A. G. Du Mez, physicians who worked for the U.S. Public Health Service and specialized in addiction. They characterized the demographic consequences of the Harrison Act in the following words: "Addiction is becoming more and more a vicious practice of unstable people who by their nature have abnormal cravings which impel them to take much larger doses that those which were taken by the average person who so often innocently fell victim to narcotics some years ago. Normal people now do not become addicted or are, as a rule, quickly cured, leaving as addicts an abnormal type with a large appetite and little means of satisfying it" (Kolb & Du Mez, 1981/1924). Kolb and Du Mez do not define key terms, such as "normal" and "unstable," but from histories of this period it is clear that they are responding to the disappearance of the middle-class laudanum drinkers.

The story of opiate use in the United States prior to the Harrison Act is consistent with current trends and practices. It should, however, be read with some reservations, since the factual sources are limited to scattered reports by those directly or indirectly involved with drug users and the distribution of drugs. Nevertheless, with decreasing degrees of certainty, the following conclusions hold. First, the connection between criminal activity and addictive drug use predates the legislative prohibitions. Second, the first few generations of American addicts prompted physicians to find a cure and legislators to issue a ban. Third, when opiates and cocaine became widely available, addiction increased, but there was not an overwhelming epidemic. These findings tell us that the labels "disease" and "criminal activity" do not fully capture the nature of addiction, although perhaps both apply to some degree. Interestingly, they suggest that there were nonlegislative and nonmedical processes at play that discouraged drug use. Opiates and cocaine were available, yet most people ignored them. The simplest explanation is that under most circumstances intoxication was not an attractive state. David Courtwright's addiction prevalence estimates (1982) say that the vast majority of nineteenth-century Americans preferred their daily routines to altered states of consciousness. The nineteenth-century demographic trends also help explain why drug use is treated both as a crime and as a symptom of disease. Opium smoking and heroin sniffing attracted a disproportionate number of unemployed youth and various delinquents. Opium eating seems to have attracted a disproportionate number of individuals who sought medical help and were seen by others as needing help. These two trends are with us today. For at least the last thirty years, men in prison comprise the population with the highest addiction rates (e.g., Anthony & Helzer, 1991), and, as discussed in Chapter 4, addicts in treatment are much more likely to have additional medical disorders than the general population (and also more nondrug medical problems than addicts who are not in treatment).

A comment regarding sentencing practices for drug offenses is in order. As noted, the manner in which the Harrison Act was enforced transformed the demographics of opiate use (Courtwright 1982; Musto, 1973). The fear of being arrested drove many users to quit or to go to considerable lengths to keep their drug habit a secret (Courtwright et al., 1989). The actual probability that possession would result in incarceration is not known with any certainty, however. Today, it is popularly believed that our prisons are filled with inmates whose only crime is using an illegal drug. On the basis of 1997 Bureau of Justice records, Jonathan Caulkins and Eric Sevigny (2005), experts on crime and drugs, checked whether this was true. Their analysis revealed that the vast majority of those in prison for drug offenses had not been locked up for possession alone. Typically, they were involved in selling illegal drugs. For example, among the drug offenders, about 2 to 15 percent were incarcerated for possession alone, with the actual figure probably closer to 2, and virtually none were in prison for possession per se if they did not have a previous record. These results are important in terms of understanding law enforcement practices, but they do not blunt the key points of this chapter. Although incarceration rates for drug possession alone may have decreased in recent years, it is still the case that possession of an illegal drug is perceived as an illegal activity and can set in motion a host of penalties, including getting fired, loss of professional privileges, loss of scholarships, and mandatory testing and counseling. Addicts who come to the attention of legal authorities may not go to prison, but there is a good chance they will lose their job and even the opportunity to pursue their livelihood. These consequences are built into various occupational and other institutional codes of conduct. In contrast, the symptoms of other psychiatric disorders do not initiate institutionalized penalties. Under a wide range of conditions, someone who is depressed or has a phobic fear of spiders does not have to worry also about automatic repercussions from his or her employer or other community institutions. Thus, even though most judges will probably hesitate to send someone to prison for drug possession, addiction remains the only psychiatric syndrome whose symptoms are illegal and automatically trigger costly punishments, which sometimes include time behind bars.

That current policies have nineteenth-century precedents does not mean that legal prohibitions should continue to be maintained or that the view that addiction is a disease is correct. History does not reveal the best drug policy or explain why people continue to inject themselves with heroin despite the realization that heroin is undermining much of what they hold valuable. These issues require a greater understanding of psychology, the brain, and the conditions that promote and inhibit drug use. These topics, particularly the conditions that inhibit drug use in addicts, are taken up in the subsequent chapters. The findings are consistent with the historical events but also add much that is new.

Addiction's Toll on American Society

What is the scope of the problem of addiction today? In the remaining pages of this chapter, I describe what happens when drugs take precedence over familial responsibilities, estimate the overall prevalence of addiction, and assess its dollar costs for taxpayers.

A personal account. The toll that addiction takes on society can be measured in terms of how drug use has hurt others, as well as by prevalence statistics and taxpayer dollars. The following story is told by a young woman whose father is identified as an addict. Her story of her childhood gives some sense of what happens when drugs come before family. The source is StoryCorps, an ongoing oral history project, initiated by Dave Isay. He was motivated by the belief that we can learn from one another's lives, that people make a difference by telling their stories to others, and that the stories are not only personal but provide a portrait of societal trends. The StoryCorps approach is simple. Two people enter a recording booth, and one, say a daughter or best friend, asks the other to tell his or her story. The process, according to the project's mission statement, "reminds us of the importance of listening to and learning from those around us. It celebrates our shared humanity. It tells people that their lives matter and they won't be forgotten." Elsewhere the StoryCorps Web site notes that stories, although personal, are of historical and social importance. The following is an excerpt that was broadcast on National Public Radio's *Morning Edition* program on June 1, 2007. LaKeisha is interviewing her best friend, Tia:

> "Who is important in your life right now?"
> "My mother, because my mother was the one that raised me, and we went through so many things together when I was little. We didn't have that much money, and whatever money we had, my father would take the money and go buy drugs, or something like that. And my mother would have to hop the subway turnstile to go to work, and she would have no money to get back."

"Did you ever get angry at your dad for being addicted to drugs?"

"I never knew him. He left when I was like one."

"Did you know anything good about him?"

"No. The only thing good I heard about him was that he came to—I think it was—my second birthday party. And after that, I've never seen him again."

"What is your father's name?"

"I don't know . . ."

"Do you think you would ever ask your mom?"

"I don't know if I should. I don't like to bring back memories from her past, because she's doing so much better now . . . Sometimes I am curious if he does wonder what I am doing, where I am. Sometimes, I wonder if he is alive or if he is dead. Some people when they get older and they never knew their birth fathers, they look for them. I don't know I would ever be able to get up the strength to really get out there and really find him. Because if I really do find him, I don't know what I would do—say, 'Hi, I'm your daughter?' And then what?"

According to LaKeisha and Tia's conversation, addiction is one of the reasons that Tia's father failed to help raise her. We do not know if Tia's father would have helped out if he had not been addicted to drugs, or if this story is representative of other addicts. However, data presented in subsequent chapters show that Tia's story does reflect trends in the empirical literature.

Prevalence and cost in dollars. Tia's story is one of millions. We can't be sure that each one is accompanied by the disappointment and hurt that Tia has experienced, but likely most do. What can be measured are prevalence rates and monetary costs. The numbers are huge and, as does Tia's story, call for a remedy. Addiction is one of America's most prevalent psychiatric disorders. According to the largest survey of psychiatric disorders on record, conducted in 2001 and 2002, almost 14 percent of Americans who are 18 years old or older have a history of addiction (Stinson et al., 2005). Approximately 12.5 percent were addicted to alcohol, almost 3 percent were addicted to an illicit drug, and between 1 and

2 percent were addicted to both. If drug abuse, which is not as serious a disorder as drug dependence, is included, the prevalence rates jump much higher. Approximately 30 percent of Americans have a history of alcohol abuse or alcohol dependence, and about 10 percent have a history of drug abuse or drug dependence (Conway et al., 2006; Hasin et al., 2007). In absolute numbers, approximately 22.5 million Americans have a history of either drug abuse or drug dependence.[3]

Tens of millions of addicted drug users imply thousands of millions of dollars in illicit drug sales. In the year 2000, Americans spent more than 64 billion dollars on illicit addictive drugs (or more than $350 for every person 18 years old or older).[4] At about the same time the government spent about 12 billion dollars on treatment and judicial programs that tried to stop these sales (ONDCP, 2004). These costs, although staggeringly large, are not the full story. Federal funds are also spent on controlling drug-related criminal activity and treating drug-related diseases.

Jonathan Caulkins and Peter Reuter (2006) point out that in the 2008, U.S. jails will house more than a "half-million drug prisoners." This is about ten times as many as in 1980. Simply maintaining this many prisoners will cost the taxpayer billions of dollars. A recent *New York Times* article puts the price tag for prison room and board at 12 billion dollars (Liptak, 2008). The Centers for Disease Control and Prevention estimated that approximately one-quarter of the 1 million HIV/AIDS cases had been transmitted by needles used to inject illegal drugs (Centers for Disease Control and Prevention, 2006). When the costs for prevention, treatment, criminal justice expenses, and lost productivity were added together for the year 2000, the total came to approximately 180 billion dollars.[5] This amounts to more than $900 for every person in the United States 18 years old and older. These costs mark an increase over previous years and are almost certainly greater today.

These estimates, although based on expert opinion, e.g., the White House drug czar's published analyses (e.g., ONDCP, 2001), include much guesswork. For example, it is not clear how to estimate "lost productivity," particularly for a population that includes many individuals who left school early and have a spotty employment record. However, even if the numbers are off, they show that addiction is a substantial drain on public resources.

These vast expenditures go hand-in-hand with large bureaucracies. Accordingly, addiction is the only psychiatric disorder that has its own federal institute. In fact it has two: the National Institute on Drug Abuse (NIDA) and the National Institute on Alcohol Abuse and Alcoholism (NIAAA). There are no national institutes on schizophrenia or phobia. Finally, addiction is the only entry in the *DSM* associated with both an actual and a metaphorical military action: the invasion of Panama to capture the then president and drug trafficker, Manuel Noriega, and the "War on Drugs."

Has the investment paid off? The magnitude of America's response to addictive drugs and addiction is reminiscent of earlier large-scale national efforts, such as the Grand Coulee Dam or Panama Canal. These projects have much to show for the expense and effort. Can the same be said for the war against drugs?

There are a number of reasonable ways to measure trends in illicit drug use. I chose "thirty-day prevalence," which is the percentage of Americans who report that they used one or more illicit drugs one or more times in the thirty days prior to responding to the survey questionnaire. The advantages of the thirty-day rates are that they are published yearly by the National Household Survey on Drug Abuse (e.g., Substance Abuse and Mental Health Services Administration, 1995, 2003, 2006), they capture first-time, regular, and heavy drug users, and as they change, so does the prevalence of addiction and other drug-related problems (e.g., Warner et al., 1995) It also should be pointed out that the National Household Survey enrolls tens of thousands of informants each year, that the interviews are conducted, supervised, and analyzed by highly experienced epidemiologists, and that the findings are widely accepted as an accurate reflection of important trends in drug use in the United States.

Figure 1.1 shows the thirty-day use trends over the years 1990 to 2005 for the most widely used illicit drugs. On the horizontal axis is the year, and on the vertical axis is the percentage of respondents who reported using an illicit drug in the thirty days prior to their interview.[6] The top panel shows the results for the highest risk group, late adolescents and young adults; the bottom panel shows the results for individuals who are less likely to use illicit drugs, those who are 26 years old and older. For all drugs and all age groups, illicit drug consumption held steady from 1990 to 2000 and then increased until 2005, when the study ended. The largest increases were for marijuana and unauthorized prescription drugs, but

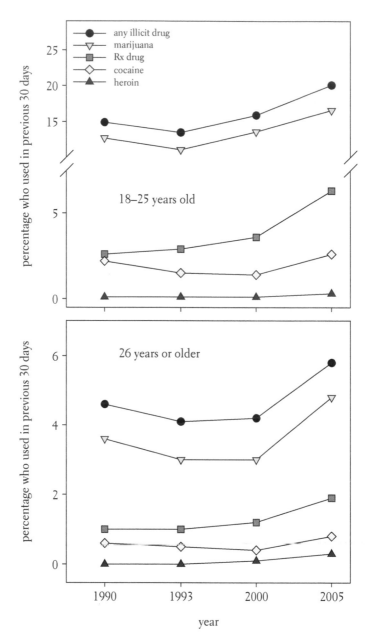

1.1 The prevalence of recent drug use (previous thirty days) as a function of year, from 1990 to 2005, and age. Recent drug use is correlated with regular drug use and addiction. Data were provided by the National Survey on Drug Use and Health.

cocaine showed slight increases as well, and heroin use remained more or less unchanged.

Given the magnitude of the support for enforcement of antidrug legislation and the remarkable recent advances in the understanding of drug and brain interactions, it is reasonable to expect a decrease in overall illicit drug use. Possibly the problem is intractable, or possibly the effort has been less effective than it could have been because of basic ideas regarding addiction. For instance, if addiction differs in significant ways from chronic disease, then treatment strategies that are successful with chronic disease are unlikely to be as successful with addiction. And of course the same logic applies to the criminal justice approach. If time in jail turns out not to increase the relative value of activities that compete with drug use, then the criminal justice approach will have little lasting influence.

Figure 1.1 provides a global overview and is a better measure of efforts to prevent the onset of illegal drug use and the transition from use to dependence. There have been many innovative programs over this same time period that have developed successful methods for reducing drug use. These include treatment programs that offer a valued gift or privilege in exchange for evidence of abstinence (described in Chapters 2 and 5) and drug courts in which the judicial system offers release from jail in exchange for abstinence (e.g., Krebs et al., 2007). These innovations borrow from both a legislative and treatment approach to addiction. However, they do not yet have a prevention counterpart.

The Current Understanding of Addiction

Although the idea that addiction is a disease had little influence outside of medicine in the nineteenth and most of the twentieth centuries, and although drug offenses are still punished by jail terms, the idea that addiction is a disease is now the prevailing view among researchers, clinicians, and the media. In clinical texts and articles, addiction is introduced as a "chronic illness" that should be classified with diseases like asthma and diabetes (e.g., Mack et al., 2003; McLellan et al., 2000; O'Brien & McLellan, 1996). In the bulletins, presentations, and articles that federal health institutes provide to schools, community groups, and the public, addiction is framed as a "chronic, relapsing, brain disease." For instance, the title of a recent National Institute on Drug Abuse (NIDA) community service slide show is "Addiction: It's a brain disease beyond a reasonable doubt" (NIDA, n.d.). The media, taking their lead from the health institute spokespersons, routinely describe addiction in these terms. In the companion book to the Home Box Office (HBO) television documentary on current scientific understandings of addiction (simply titled *Addiction*), which aired in 2007, one chapter is titled, "Addiction Is a Brain Disease" and another is titled, "A Disease of Young People" (Hoffman & Froemke, 2007).

My impression is that the journalists' presentations resonate with the public. People who have nothing at stake other than being well-informed agree that addiction is a disease. In chance encounters, I find that most people believe that the disease interpretation of addiction is the scientific, enlightened, and humane perspective. As ideas are usually understood in terms of general, pre-existing beliefs, that both experts and nonexperts have so readily embraced the disease interpretation of addiction suggests that it fits well with what most people already think about drugs and human motives. This idea is explored further in Chapter 5 in the context of the conceptual and factual basis for current understandings of addiction.

Although the ability to hold opposing ideas in mind at once is said to have its advantages, resolving the contradictions attending addiction has advantages too. It is not fair to punish some and offer to cure others who exhibit the same behaviors. These inequities are quite likely joined by inefficiencies. If treating addiction is the right approach, then punishing addicts for drug use has to be at least somewhat ineffective, if not counterproductive. Conversely, if punishing drug use is the right approach, then treatment programs that do not offer or facilitate differential consequences for abstinence are likely to be less effective than they could be. Put more generally, it seems unlikely that approaches that are as different as punishment and treatment effectively complement one another. This in turn suggests that some portion of the billions of dollars that are spent on these two approaches could be spent more wisely. Common sense says that the first step toward a more effective and efficient response to addiction is to formulate a coherent, research-based account of its nature.

To this end, I have found it useful to address a series of questions on the relationship between drug use and biology, drug use and the individual, and drug use and society. Chapter 2 addresses when, why, and where addiction first appeared. Chapter 4 addresses whether addiction is really a chronic disorder, where "chronic" is understood to imply at least ten or so years of heavy drug use. Chapter 3 asks what addiction is like when the addicts themselves are describing their lives. Most of what we learn about addiction is from experts. Do the addicts agree with the experts? Chapter 5 addresses the question of whether addiction's biological basis, which is well established, implies that it is a disease. It is widely held that a genetic predisposition for addiction and drug-induced neural adaptations make addiction a disease. Is this a sensible interpretation of these relationships? Chapter 6 addresses a general question that pertains to addiction as well as other forms of voluntary yet self-destructive action. How is it possible for individuals to pursue ends that are on balance self-defeating? The question is relevant to psychology in general and to the various accounts of human behavior that assume that choice is rational. The last chapter uses the findings of Chapter 6 to address the question of what makes a substance addictive and why some individuals are more likely than others to use drugs self-destructively.

One of the assumptions that influences discussions of the nature of addiction is that the disease interpretation is the most humane or sympathetic position, one which will lead to more effective treatment programs (e.g., Miller & Chappel, 1991). The reasoning behind this view is that if addiction is a disease, then science will soon find an effective treatment for it, as has been the case for many other diseases, but that if addiction is a matter of choice, then the appropriate response is punishment. For example, if people are choosing to harm themselves and their activity also harms others, then they are getting what they deserve and the damage to society calls for a righting of the scales of justice and retribution. The core assumption in this viewpoint is that there are but two possible responses to addiction: medical treatment or punishment. This way of thinking informed the discussion of addiction by physicians in the late nineteenth century and continues to inform the discussion of treatment options today. Dr. Norman Kerr, who was mentioned earlier as an early promoter of the disease interpretation, contrasted his medical-disease approach to the "dark ages when inebriates were viewed as 'vicious depraved sinners'" (Berridge, 1990). About one hundred years later, Alan Leshner, director of NIDA during the 1990s, offered readers of *Science* the same two choices (1997): "The gulf in implications between the 'bad person' view and the 'chronic illness' sufferer view is tremendous. As just one example there are many people who believe that addicted individuals do not deserve treatment."

What needs to be pointed out is that medical treatment and punishment do not exhaust the possible responses to human problems. We teach, offer advice, arrange contingencies, and in general have a wide array of techniques for improving social relations and the behavior of others. To take but one example relevant to addiction, choice-oriented clinicians and researchers have developed programs that teach addicts to take advantage of nondrug alternatives (e.g., Higgins et al., 2000; Silverman et al., 1996). These programs are considered among the most effective approaches for getting addicts off drugs. They fit neither a medical nor penal model of rehabilitation. Rather, they are the most logical treatment approach if addiction is not a compulsive disorder but one in which voluntary behavior is self-destructive. If a choice process drives drug use in addiction, then it is in principle possible to arrange conditions such that addicts will be persuaded to choose something other than intoxication. This approach involves neither medicine nor punishment. Alcoholics Anonymous (AA) and other popular twelve-step treatments are not really medical programs either. They produce positive outcomes by enhancing the value of activities that compete with drug use and have developed effective techniques for encouraging hope in a brighter future. Their techniques are not what students learn in medical school or criminology graduate school, yet, as I describe in Chapter 7, AA works.

The next chapter addresses the question of when and where addiction first appeared. Did the discovery of opiates lead, lockstep, to a new phenomenon, opiate addiction? This question is a specific instance of a more general issue: What are the necessary and sufficient conditions for addiction? Exposure to even the most addictive drugs does not necessarily lead to addiction, but it is not clear what other factors play a role. For example, there appears to be an emerging consensus that addiction is an equal-opportunity disease, meaning that demographic factors such as poverty, low educational attainment, and neighborhood play little or no role in differences in the likelihood of drug use graduating to drug abuse (e.g., Hoffman & Froemke, 2007; Rosenberg et al., 1995). As we will see, though, there are well-established published research reports that suggest a somewhat different picture.

2

THE FIRST DRUG EPIDEMIC

Most people who use addictive drugs do not become addicted to them. Almost everyone has had at least one alcoholic drink and a healthy percentage of the population drinks alcohol regularly, yet most people are not alcoholics. Similarly, many people have experimented with marijuana, cocaine, opiates, and stimulants, yet only a minority go on to become addicted to these drugs. Although it is obvious that the percentage of addicts is dwarfed by the percentage of those who could be addicts, the observation is puzzling. Drugs act on neurons, and everyone's neurons function in the same way. Indeed, neurons function in nearly identical ways across the entire animal kingdom. Heroin binds to *mu* opioid receptor sites in humans, chimpanzees, and rats. If experimentation with heroin can lead to heroin addiction in one person, and heroin functions in pretty much the same way in everyone's nervous system, then why doesn't everyone who uses heroin become a heroin addict?

These observations reveal a well-established psychopharmacological principle. The behavioral effects of drugs vary as a function of the setting and the individual. An interesting study on social relations in monkeys showed that stimulants increased aggression, particularly in the dominant monkey, but the degree to which they did so varied as a function of the monkey's personality and current place in the troop hierarchy (e.g., Martin et al., 1990). Similarly, alcohol increases gregariousness as well as aggression depending on individual differences and local conditions (e.g., Steele & Josephs, 1990). In psychopharmacology articles and books, these and similar observations therefore prompt the statement "drug effects depend on the setting and the individual." While true, the summary seems to do little more than reiterate the observations. What is missing is an account of how it is possible for individual differences and setting to alter the manner in which powerful drugs alter behavior. For instance, social status emerges at the level of social interactions, so how can it influence the manner in which a drug alters behavior? The actual physical, mechanical interactions are far from obvious. The last section of this chapter takes up this problem. It offers a general account of how setting, including such ephemera as religion and cultural values, could, in principle, alter the course of drug effects and addiction. The account is based on the structure of the nervous system and the idea that at the neuronal level, drug effects and ideas take the same physical form. Values, experience, and receptor binding all influence how neurons behave, and a fundamental property of neurons is to influence each other. Thus, personal values and economic options can affect the consequences of drug use (e.g., receptor binding) at the level of neuronal interactions.

First, however, some of the key findings regarding the likelihood that drug use leads to drug addiction will be described. This story begins with the history of opiate use and the emergence of the first drug "epidemic." This will be followed by some basic epidemiological findings that apply to current conditions. The results reveal that one of the most important etiological factors in addiction is the immediate social environment.

Historical Origins of Opium Use

Of the drugs that are currently prohibited by law, opiates were the first to be used recreationally by large numbers of people and the first to be outlawed. For millennia opium was a medical remedy, but when it began to be used as an intoxicant, it lost its universal acclaim. The menacing John Jasper in Charles Dickens's last novel, *The Mystery of Edwin Drood* (1870), is an opium habitué, and in Oscar Wilde's *The Picture of Dorian Gray* (1890), the opium den is home to those who have lost their moral compass.

Opium at the dawn of written history. Opium is extracted from the seed capsule of a lovely species of flowering annual poppy, *Papaver somniferum*—literally "sleep inducing poppy." At maturity, its petals fall off, leaving a bulbous seed pod. The seed pod contains a latex-like substance that can be extracted by scoring the pod's tough skin. The sap contains morphine and codeine, the plant's primary active ingredients.

The earliest evidence linking the opium plant and humans is fossilized, charred poppy seed cakes found among the litter of European settlements from the Neolithic period (4800–2600 BC; Merlin, 1984). In the absence of written and iconographic records, it cannot be known for certain whether these early Europeans used the opium poppy for its medicinal and mind-altering properties. However, given that the seeds were ingested and the morphine-rich sap is so easy to access, nonnutritional uses seem likely.

Bronze Age (1600–1200 BC) artifacts provide the earliest definitive evidence that the opium poppy was cultivated for its curative and psychotropic properties. Ancient Greek relics display representations of the seed capsule in association with Nyx, Hypnos, Morpheus, and Asclepius, the gods of the night, sleep, dreams, and medicine. In Greek myths and Homer's epic poems, opium plays its now familiar role as a narcotic. Theseus put Cerberus, the many-headed dog that guards Hades, to sleep with opium. In the *Iliad*, Helen mixes "nepenthe" with wine to help the survivors of the Trojan War forget their sorrows. Nepenthe is almost certainly a reference to opium. The Ebers Papyrus, one of the earliest written documents in existence (ca. 1550 BC), includes a description of plant seeds and plant capsules that are particularly useful for soothing crying infants and headaches. The description fits the opium poppy better than any other known plant.

The chroniclers of ancient Greece and Egypt always showed opium in a positive light. They emphasized its medicinal value and psychological benefits. It provided relief from pain, sorrow, and disease. In contrast to later accounts, the ancient sources did not portray opium as a danger to the individual or society. This was not self-censorship. Greek and Roman essayists were not shy to scold their fellow citizens for excessive drinking. That there were no similar scolds for opium suggests that they had nothing bad to say about it.

Opiates in the Middle Ages and Renaissance. The image of opium as a healthful elixir persists for millennia, and if anything grows stronger. For instance, some three thousand years after the authors of the Ebers Papyrus jotted down how to cure colic, the author of a major sixteenth-century medical text, Paracelsus (1493–1541), referred to tinctures of opium as "laudanum"—an object worthy of praise—and "the stone of immortality," extending life. Writing in the seventeenth century, Thomas Sydenham (1624–1689), who is sometimes described as the father of English medicine, echoes Paracelsus' views: "among the remedies which it has pleased Almighty God to give to man to relieve his sufferings, none is so universal and so efficacious as opium." So, for the first three thousand years or so of written history, opium is not simply one of many medicines used by healers, it is nature's most efficacious elixir and the most heralded.[1]

Recreational opiate use in China. Although the early history of opium is largely European, addiction appears first in China. A key player in the history of opium is the spread of tobacco. European sailors discovered tobacco smoking on their voyages to the New World. The natives "drank smoke," they reported back home. "Smoking," as it came to be known, proved popular in Europe and everywhere the sailors traveled. When European sailors introduced the Chinese to tobacco, they too took to smoking. They used pipes as did the sixteenth-century European navigators, but in contrast to other cultures, the Chinese began to add opium to the tobacco. This is significant because smoking delivers the active component of opium, morphine, to the brain much more rapidly than ingesting it orally. And the faster the rate of delivery of a drug, the more concentrated the dose at its sites of action.[2]

Opium smoking spread rapidly in China, giving rise to new smoking paraphernalia and special places to smoke, the notorious opium dens. This is the first known instance of large numbers of people taking opium for its intoxicating effects rather than its medical effects (Latimer & Goldberg, 1981; Spence, 1975). With these changes, the public image of opium changed. It was no longer a gift from Providence; it was a scourge. A Chinese soldier's diary entry preserved from the year 1724 claims that those who smoked opium were foolish and delinquent (cited in Spence, 1975): "Opium smoking was a harmful trap, set by Barbarians to ensnare 'Han Chinese.' The uninitiated were given free opium at first, but once they were hooked, they were made to pay. The smokers are gullible and criminal." Set against the record of the previous three millennia, this is a remarkable passage. Opium had been revered as a gift from God and one of nature's gifts to mankind. With the onset of recreational opium smoking, it becomes a trap and an accessory to those who are foolish and delinquent.

This diarist was not the only one alarmed by opium smoking. In 1725 the emperor of China issued an edict outlawing the sale of opium. The edict proved unenforceable. Three-quarters of a century later, in 1799, a second imperial anti-opium edict was issued. It listed more severe penalties than the first and was accompanied by an explanation for why opium should be outlawed. The Jiaqing Emperor is quoted as follows (in Latimer & Goldberg, 1981):

> The use of opium originally prevailed only among vagrants and disreputable persons . . . but has since extended itself among the members and descendants of respectable families, students, and officers of the government. When this habit becomes established by frequent repetition, it gains an entire ascendence, and the consumer of opium is not only unable to forbear from its daily use, but on passing the accustomed hour, cannot refrain from tears or command himself in any degree. The extraordinary expense of this article is likewise to be noticed . . . which the fortunes of the bulk of the community are unable to satisfy, and are therefore wholly dilapidated and wasted.

Although the emperor's observations are more than two hundred years old, his remarks describe addiction as it is understood today. He points out that opiate smoking was originally a practice favored by "disreputable people" that has now spread to proper, otherwise law-abiding citizens, that it squeezes out important interests so that it comes to dominate all other activities, and that if opium is not taken regularly, uncomfortable withdrawal symptoms ensue, which further increases the hold that the drug has on the helpless "consumer." But the harm is not just to the smoker. The emperor recognizes that the economics of addiction set in motion a downward spiral that saps the user, his family, and his community of their wealth.[3]

What explains the emergence of opiate addiction in China? The written record shows that for three thousand years, opiates had been used without incident or at least without incident worthy of reporting. The archeological and botanical evidence pushes these dates back by an additional two millennia. But even five thousand years of trouble-free benefits may be an underestimate. Given how easy it is to tap the narcotic sap of the opium poppy, it is reasonable to suppose that humans have been taking advantage of the plant's medicinal benefits for eons. As soon as smoking became an established practice, however, opium addiction became a problem. The culprit, or more accurately, one of the culprits, is a change in pharmacological action. The lungs deliver opium's active components to the brain much more rapidly than does the stomach, thereby increasing its concentration at the sites of action.

The shift from oral self-administration to smoking plays a critical role in the first addiction epidemic, but a quicker onset of action could not have been the only factor. The Chinese were but one of many peoples who took up smoking in the seventeenth and eighteenth centuries, and the British were eager to trade opium with everyone. India and Britain did not witness large increases in the demand for opium, yet India was where most of the commercial opium was grown, and the British were the traffickers. Why, then, did the first opium epidemic occur just in China when it could have occurred in so many other countries? Scholars have yet to address this question. It is possible to outline, albeit somewhat speculatively, the general form of the answer. The additional factors are societal, historical, and possibly genetic.

The societal factors include surplus wealth and available leisure time. Smoking opium takes up a good deal of time and requires disposable income. This predicts that relative to other countries, eighteenth-century China had a disproportionately large number of individuals with time on their hands, individuals with disposable income, and individuals in a position to trade with the British. Likely candidates are the regional war lords, imperial palace civil servants, government bureaucrats, the large standing army that existed in China, and the various personages who reaped the benefits of the agricultural surpluses. Changes in laudanum consumption support this interpretation. In England in the seventeenth century laudanum was a medicine. At the end of the nineteenth century, the British considered it an addictive drug and took measures to control its distribution. This change corresponds to an increase in upper-class laudanum habitués, individuals who had both money and leisure time, and the emergence of a working class who had some disposable income, some of which they spent on opiates (e.g., Berridge, 1997).

Historical and genetic differences may have also paved the way for a particular fondness for opium in China. In Europe in the Middle Ages, opium was known largely for its medicinal value. In China in the Middle Ages, opium served an important additional purpose. It was a popular aphrodisiac. Thus, prior to the onset of smoking there was a recreational aspect to opium that existed in China but not the West. Last, China may also have been home to a pent-up demand for intoxication that had genetic roots. Many Chinese have a toxic reaction to alcohol (e.g., Luczak et al., 2001). Alcohol makes them sick, and the cause is an inability to rapidly metabolize a poisonous metabolite of alcohol (acetaldehyde). If we assume that individuals, particularly those living in societies undergoing change, value intoxication, then opium may have been more valued by the Chinese than other peoples because they did not have alcohol as an alternative. The inability to take advantage of alcohol's intoxicating properties may also explain why the Chinese were more likely to ascribe aphrodisiacal properties to opium than were Europeans.

Although these additional social, historical, and genetic explanations are speculative, they rest on solid ground. Since smoking was a world-wide practice and the British and peoples of India had easier access to opium than did the Chinese, pharmacology could not have been the only factor in the emergence of the opium problem in China. The logical possibilities are social, historical, and individual, and there is circumstantial evidence that each played a role.

The Probability that Drug Use Turns into Drug Abuse

"It's so good you only have to try it once" applies to heroin, not alcohol or tobacco. One of the implications of this saying is that drugs that are prohibited are more addictive than those that are legal. This seems reasonable, but measuring "addictiveness" is problematic. A law-abiding citizen may crave heroin, but because he is afraid of being arrested, he smokes a cigarette or has a drink, which he considers second- and third-best alternatives. Given these considerations, a reasonable although clearly imperfect approach is to calculate the likelihood that drug use leads to drug addiction for drugs that have roughly similar socially mediated consequences. This measure controls for exposure in that it applies only to those who have ever used a particular drug. Thus, to the degree that other consequences can be equated, it measures pharmacological differences. Of course, other consequences cannot really be made equal, but the results are nevertheless of interest. For instance, over the last forty or so years, cocaine has replaced heroin as the prototypical drug of abuse. Cocaine also conveys less stigma than does heroin, so that for a variety of reasons, we should predict that cocaine use is more likely than heroin use to lead to addiction. There are published data that allow us to calculate the probabilities, but before we look at the answers, there is a methodological matter that cannot be ignored, either in this book or in any study of addiction. This is who counts as an "addict."

According to researchers and clinicians an addict is someone who fits the criteria for "substance dependence" in the American Psychiatric Association's (APA) *Diagnostic and Statistical Manual of Mental Disorders* (APA, 1994). This is also the approach taken in virtually all of the studies that contributed to this book, and for good reason. The criteria have proven reliable and valid.[4] Different raters usually agree as to who is and is not an addict, and those who meet the *DSM* criteria differ from those who do not as measured by demographic, psychological, and biological indices.[5] However, the *DSM* uses the term "substance dependence," not "addiction." So we need to ask if the two terms refer to the same phenomenon.

"Addiction" and *"substance dependence."* In everyday speech, self-destructive drug users are called "addicts." According to the *DSM* they are "substance dependent." The different words raise the possibility that perhaps addiction and substance dependence are different. Several lines of evidence reveal that they are synonyms.

First, according to *DSM* nomenclature, substance dependence is the most extreme form of self-destructive drug use. Similarly, according to everyday usage, drug addiction is the most extreme form of self-destructive drug use.

Second, substance dependence is identified by the classic symptoms of addiction, such as tolerance, withdrawal, relapse, and a shift in priorities in favor of the drug. The exact words are (APA, 1994): "The essential feature of Substance Dependence is a cluster of cognitive, behavioral, and physiological symptoms indicating that the individual continues use of the substance despite significant substance-related problems. There is a pattern of repeated self-administration that usually results in tolerance, withdrawal, and compulsive drug-taking behavior" (p. 176). Following this passage is a list of seven observable, measurable signs related to drug use, such as tolerance, withdrawal, using more drug than initially intended or failing to stop using after vowing to do so. If three or more of these symptoms are present in the previous twelve months, then the drug user is considered drug dependent.

Third, the *DSM* defines substance dependence as "compulsive" drug use. In a similar vein, dictionaries define "drug addiction" as compulsive drug use (e.g., *Oxford English Dictionary*). Thus, the signs of "substance dependence" and "addiction" are the same and the interpretation of the signs are the same: those who are substance dependent, or "addicts," are compulsive drug users. This of course does not mean that "compulsive" is the proper interpretation, but it is one that academics and the public can agree upon. We can be assured then that when researchers talk about "substance dependence," they are also talking about "addiction."

Drug use and addiction in the United States. Figures 2.1 and 2.2 show the prevalence and addiction rates for the most common illicit drugs and for alcohol. They are based on interviews conducted in 2001 and 2002. The subjects are representative of the country as a whole according to ethnicity, residence, income, education, gender, and other demographic measures. One study (SAMHSA) recruited approximately 67,000 subjects; the other, the National Epidemiologic Survey on Alcohol and Related Conditions (NESARC), recruited approximately 43,000 subjects.[6] The data shown here are for subjects aged 18 years and older.

Figure 2.1 shows that about half the informants had used an illicit drug one or more times. About 45 percent reported using marijuana; about 2 percent reported using an opiate. The percentages for other illicit drugs

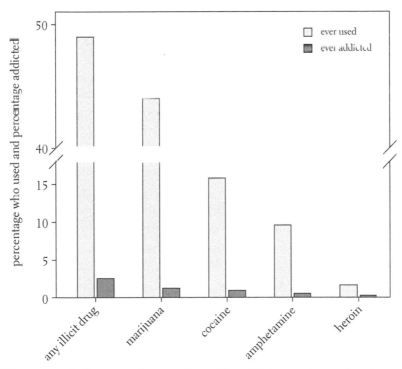

2.1 Lifetime use and addiction as a function of type of drug. Lifetime use data are from the 2002 National Survey on Drug Use and Health (SAMHSA, 2003); lifetime addiction percentages are from the National Epidemiologic Survey on Alcohol and Related Conditions (NESARC) (Conway et al., 2006).

fall in between these two extremes. The darkest bars show those who met the *DSM* criteria for addiction, either currently or in the past. That these bars are so much shorter means that most people who used did not become addicted. For example, about 50 percent of the informants reported that they had used an illicit drug at least once, whereas according to the interviews, less than 3 percent of informants have a history of dependence on an illicit drug. About half the addiction cases involved marijuana, and the other half involved either stimulants or opiates.

The percentages may seem small, but as measured in number of lives they are large. In the year 2000 there were more than 210 million Americans who were 18 years or older, so that at the time of the survey there were close to 6 million current and ex–drug addicts. To gain some perspective on what this means, the number of addicts is about the same as the population of a mid-size state, for example Tennessee, and is about twice as large as that of the 101 towns and cities that make up the Greater Boston area. This is a lot of heavy, self-destructive drug users, enough to produce the harm and expense documented in the previous chapter.

Figure 2.2 shows the likelihood that drug use led to addiction (i.e., the addiction rates) for the most widely used illicit drugs and for alcohol. The results reflect differences in pharmacology, differences in the populations that are attracted to the different drugs, and differences in the conditions that surround drug use. For example, the figure shows opiate addiction rates for Americans at home and American enlistees in Vietnam during the Vietnam War.

The U.S. opiate addiction rate was almost seven times higher than the marijuana addiction rate, even though the sanctions and stigma associated with opiates are much greater. This suggests that opiates are much more addictive. The differences in the U.S. and Vietnam heroin rates reflect social influences and drug availability. Enlistees who served in Vietnam reported that high quality opium and heroin were easy to come by and cheap (Robins, 1993; Robins et al., 1975, 1980). According to novels and movies (e.g., *Apocalypse Now*), not only were the drugs everywhere, but there was also little fear of punishment or even disapproval for using them. The enlistees did not have to risk going into a "bad" neighborhood to obtain illicit drugs or risk rejection from their peers. Under these conditions, the addiction rates for opiates more than doubled.

The results run counter to the expectation that illicit drug use is more likely to lead to addiction than alcohol is to lead to alcoholism. On aver-

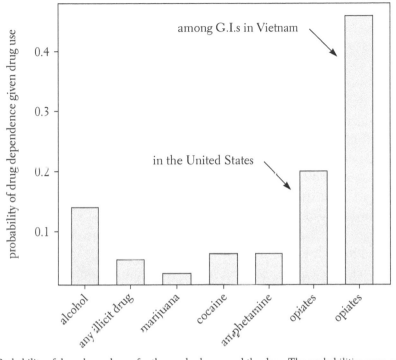

2.2 Probability of drug dependence for those who have used the drug. The probabilities were calculated on the basis of data from the previous figure. The alcohol results are from NESARC.

age about 5 percent of those who used an illicit drug became a drug addict, whereas about 15 percent of those who ever had a drink went on to become an alcoholic. Opiates, namely heroin, are the exception. About 20 percent of U.S. opiate users went on to become addicted, and about 45 percent of Vietnam enlistees who used an opiate one or more times graduated to heavy use and withdrawal symptoms.

The influence of cohort on addiction. The differences between the U.S. and Vietnam addiction rates on the one hand suggest that the etiology of addiction varies substantially as a function of societal conditions, particularly attitudes toward drugs. On the other hand, the Vietnam drug experience may not really be representative of the normal course of addiction. The enlistees were fighting an unpopular war under grueling circumstances, and against a dangerous enemy. These conditions may be so far from normal that the findings, although interesting, are idiosyncratic. If so, then it is possible that the prevalence of addiction is actually relatively stable, only varying as a function of pharmacological and individual differences. This was tested by looking at the relationship between addiction rates and year of birth (cohort). This approach takes advantage of the fact that there have been large changes in attitudes toward drug use over the last fifty years or so. In the 1960s and 1970s illicit drug use became more widely accepted than it was in earlier years. This is similar to what happened in Vietnam, albeit on a smaller scale. Thus, if social conditions influence the etiology of addiction, then the prevalence of addiction and perhaps even the likelihood that drug use leads to addiction will vary as a function of cohort.

"Cohort" is a demographic term used to identify a group of people bound by a common event, typically year of birth. For instance, sociologists assign the "Baby Boomer" cohort the birth years of about 1946 to 1964, and they allot the "Generation X" cohort the years 1965 to 1982. Cohorts differ in terms of historical influences and, of course, age. Hence, if a researcher controls for age, the cohort differences reflect historical factors (assuming no major shifts in population characteristics, such as those that result from changing immigration patterns). The National Comorbidity Survey, a nationwide study of psychiatric disorders headed by Ronald Kessler, employed just this strategy (2005a, 2005b, and Warner et al., 1995). They determined the likelihood that illicit drug use led to addiction as a function of age for four different cohorts, spanning the period 1940 to 1990. The basic finding was that cohorts born after World War II had much higher addiction rates at all ages. For example, a drug user who was 20 in 1990 (Generation X, b. 1970) was about eight times more likely to become addicted than a drug user who was 20 in 1960 (pre-"Youth Culture," pre-"Baby Boomer," b. 1940).

The major cultural difference that is directly relevant to drugs for the pre– and post–World War II cohorts is the advent of "Youth Culture" in the 1960s. Illicit drugs became commonplace at parties and concerts, a popular mantra of the day was "Tune in, turn on, drop out," and movies and television shows featured hip, attractive, smart people doing lines of cocaine for fun. It is likely that these factors were among those that led to the sharp increase in addiction rates in the more recent cohorts. However, whatever the causes, the cohort effects demonstrate that the dramatic increase in addiction rates among Vietnam enlistees was not an historical oddity. The cohort increases in the United States are considerably greater. The implication is that social conditions play an important role in the etiology of addiction.

Other disorders show cohort effects, but not nearly as large as those reported by the National Comorbidity Survey for substance dependence. The results are hard to compare, however, because the historical periods differed. The ideal way to tell if addiction is more susceptible to historical trends than other psychiatric disorders is to study the influence of cohort on different disorders in the same individuals. This way the variables are all the same except those related to the disorders. The next figure shows the results from an epidemiological study that took just this approach.

Figure 2.3 compares cohort effects for different psychiatric disorders. One cohort was born well before the start of World War II, and one born well after the end of World War II. The results were taken from tables published by the first large, scientific survey of the prevalence of psychiatric disorders in the United States—the Epidemiologic Catchment Area Study (ECA) (Robins & Regier, 1991).[7] On the horizontal axis is a list of the disorders for which cohort information was available. On the vertical axis is the percentage of interviewees who ever met the criteria for the disorder ("lifetime prevalence"). The filled black bars indicate

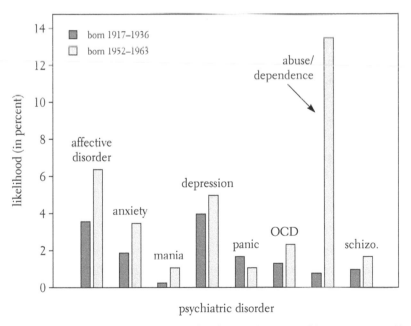

2.3 Differences in the likelihood of psychiatric disorders as a function of differences in year of birth. Drug-use disorders show the largest cohort effects. Data are from Robins & Regier, 1991.

prevalence for the earlier cohort, the open white bars show prevalence for the more recent cohort. But as age and cohort go together, the individuals in the older cohort (filled black bars) had more time to develop a disorder. Hence, all else being equal, the black bars should be as high or higher than the open white bars.

Although the older cohorts had more time to develop symptoms, the more recent cohort (and younger subjects) were more likely to report a history of psychiatric problems. However, the differences were not particularly large, except in one case. The exception was drug dependence. The likelihood of ever meeting the criteria for a substance disorder was about fifteen times higher in the post–World War II cohort. This replicates the large National Comorbidity Survey cohort effects described above. The figure also shows that cohort effects are not simply a characteristic of addiction, but that this influence differentiates addiction from all other disorders in the *DSM* for which there are historical data. As measured by cohort, addiction is a psychiatric outlier.

The most obvious interpretation of the large cohort effects for addiction is that the results are influenced by cultural trends to a greater extent than other psychiatric disorders. This is relevant to efforts to curb addiction. If changes in setting lead to dramatic increases in addiction, then it is possible that changes in setting can also lead to dramatic decreases in addiction. There are other interpretations of the cohort effects that should be considered, however.

The survey results are based on face-to-face interviews. Hence, diagnoses for disorders that are no longer present have to be reconstructed from memory. Individuals who currently do not meet diagnostic thresholds may systematically underestimate past problems. This could explain the trend for more recent cohorts to report somewhat higher lifetime prevalence rates for most psychiatric disorders. But it is not obvious why the recall effect should be so much greater for addiction. Indeed, according to the joke that "If you remember the sixties, you weren't there," the trend should be just the opposite.

Another possibility is that post–World War II generations experimented with drugs that were more addictive, namely heroin and cocaine. For instance, the addiction rate graph showed that heroin was much more likely to lead to addiction than was marijuana. But heroin addiction is rare and most likely counted for no more than a small fraction of the results summarized in Figures 2.1, 2.2, and 2.3. In support of this point, opiates counted for less than 10 percent of all instances of drug addiction in the most recent and to date the largest national epidemiological study (Conway, et al., 2006). Thus, differential drug use seems an unlikely explanation for the association between differences in cohort and differences in addiction rates.

These considerations suggest that drug availability and changes in attitudes, values, and perhaps sanctions or perceived sanctions explain the large differences. Whatever the reason, it is clear that addiction is much more subject to historical trends than other *DSM* disorders. Over periods of months and years, addiction rates changed by as much as a factor of eight.

The influence of neighborhood on drug use. In gritty television crime shows, movies, and novels, addicts live in poor, inner-city neighborhoods that are populated mostly by African Americans and Hispanics. In contrast, the cover of the book and the DVD that accompanies the 2007 HBO series on addiction shows mostly white men and women, many of whom are in jacket and tie (*Why Can't They Just Stop?* Hoffman & Froemke, 2007). The cover's message is that addiction is an equal-opportunity disorder. In support of this claim, the inside pages list twenty-two "expert contributors," none of whom discuss addiction in terms of historical trends or demographic factors that pertain to social economic status. Similarly, articles published in leading medical journals include summary statements that support the equal-opportunity version of addiction. In the *New England Journal of Medicine*, the authors of an article on drug use during pregnancy write, "the use of illicit drugs is common among pregnant women regardless of race and socioeconomic status" (Chasnoff et al., 1990), and similarly in a paper published in the *Archives of Pediatrics & Adolescent Medicine*, the authors conclude that "the geographic distribution of drug use is diverse and egalitarian" (Rosenberg et al., 1995).

Who is correct: the television shows that place addiction in the inner city, or the experts who place it everywhere? A particularly interesting set of studies that assessed the relationship between neighborhood and drug use can help us answer this question. The results are particularly valuable because drug use was determined by a biological assay rather than verbal report. Will Brownsberger (1997) summarized the finding in a paper titled, "Prevalence of frequent cocaine use in urban poverty areas."

The subjects were pregnant women and neonates, and the assays were obtained from urine and meconium samples. These samples provide valid measures of cocaine use.

Brownsberger gathered data on poor neighborhoods, defined as those in which 40 percent or more of the population met federal criteria for poverty.[8] Some neighborhoods were rural, some metropolitan, and some were in large cities. The basic finding was that the proportion of mothers who tested positive for cocaine varied systematically as a function of the type of neighborhood. Mothers from large inner-city neighborhoods were about four times more likely to test positive than mothers from smaller urban areas, and these mothers were in turn about four times more likely to test positive than mothers from poor rural areas. For inner-city hospitals, the median percentage of cocaine-positive mothers was 12 percent, and for rural hospitals it was 1 percent. Moreover, there was no overlap between the rural hospital results and the inner-city hospital results.

Figure 2.4 summarizes the results from studies conducted in neighborhoods with similar income distributions.[9] The results show that drug use varied as a function of neighborhood even when income was held constant. But what if income also varied? Figure 2.5 evaluates the issue. The top panel plots cocaine use as a function of income for pregnant women who were seen at a Rochester, New York, hospital. Income was determined by the mother's zip code. As in the studies just discussed, the investigators used the (meconium) assay to test for cocaine (Ryan et al., 1994). The bottom panel displays abuse and dependence as a function of income (Anthony & Helzer, 1991). The figure is based on tables summarizing the findings of the nationwide Epidemiologic Catchment Area Study. The results from both studies indicate that drug use and drug disorders decrease as income increases.

The analysis displayed in Figure 2.5 does not dissociate income from neighborhood, and neither study definitively establishes the causal relationships between demographic factors and drug use. But there is a matter of converging independent sources of information and simplicity. The income and neighborhood analyses reveal the same pattern of results as the analyses based on cohort; and the income, neighborhood, and cohort findings are consistent with the marked increase in opiate use and addiction among the Vietnam enlistees. The research methods included face-to-face interviews, questionnaires, and metabolic assays. Despite the disparate methods, the results were the same: the immedi-

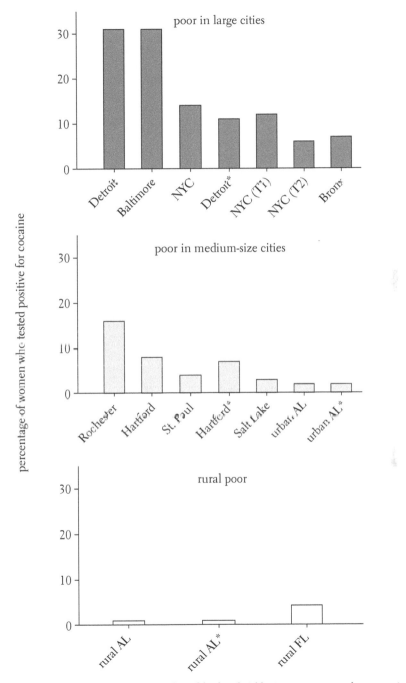

2.4 Differences in cocaine use as a function of neighborhood. Addiction is not an equal-opportunity disorder. Based on a literature review by Brownsberger, 1997.

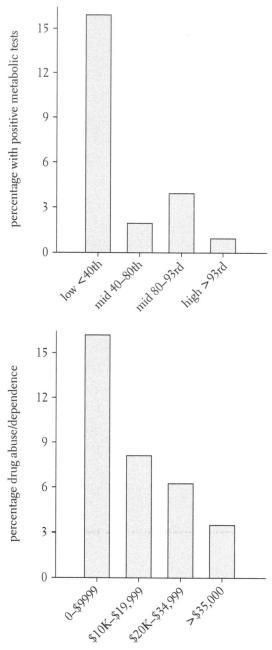

2.5 Drug use and drug disorders as a function of income. The top panel shows cocaine use as a function of income in Rochester, New York (Ryan et al., 1994). The bottom panel shows abuse and dependence as a function of income in the nationwide ECA survey (Anthony & Helzer, 1991). Income differences in drug use and dependence are not particularly large, except for the lowest income group.

ate social environment as well as nationwide cultural trends influenced the prevalence of illicit drug use and the likelihood that drug use became drug abuse. The cohort association was stronger for addiction than for any other psychiatric disorder by more than an order of magnitude (see Figure 2.3). The simplest interpretation is that social factors play an important role in the etiology of addiction and a relatively small role in the etiology of other psychiatric disorders. Addiction is not an equal-opportunity disorder; indeed there is no psychiatric disorder that is more closely tied to circumstance.

How Drugs Work

This chapter shows that differences in social circumstances have a profound influence on the likelihood that drug use escalates to drug abuse. Differences in social conditions include differences in ideas, values, and attitudes. Thus, it is reasonable to suppose that the relationship between social setting and addiction rates reflects the influence of ideas, values, and attitudes on the likelihood that drug use turns into drug abuse. In support of this inference, social settings in which addictive drugs lost some of their negative connotations witnessed dramatic increases in addiction rates (e.g., post–World War II cohorts and Vietnam). This is a puzzling result. Values and attitudes emerge in the context of individuals interacting with each other; they depend on social traditions. Drugs are biological agents that act on neurons. How can values influence drug effects? The two seem incommensurable, and as drugs are more fundamental, the manner in which values suppress and facilitate drug effects is not obvious. This issue is not unique to the results presented in this chapter but applies to all psychopharmacological research. Put most broadly, the question is, "How do psychological phenomena influence biological phenomena?" This is one of the fundamental issues in psychological research, and one in which there has been much progress in recent years. The research focuses on the central nervous system (CNS). Drugs, the environment (including social setting), and psychological phenomena affect the workings of the central nervous system. Thus, by describing basic features of the CNS, it is possible to obtain some understanding of how values and other psychological phenomena can influence drug effects. The discussion will focus on neurons because drugs act directly on neurons. The account, though, is quite general, omitting much of what has been learned in recent years about the complex interactions and various mechanisms that characterize brain functioning and the brain's response to drugs (e.g., Koob & Le Moal, 2006).

The central nervous system and drug use. The CNS mediates thought, affect, and action. It is involved in everything that we call "psychological." This has been documented in countless research projects, starting with nineteenth-century accounts of reflex arcs to today's brain-imaging studies. The relationship between the CNS and psychological phenomena is also implied by evolution. Evolutionary processes led to humans and other animals, humans and other animals behave psychologically, thus evolution implies that psychological phenomena must have a physical basis.

The CNS is a complex network made up of billions of interconnected elements called neurons. Each neuron has multiple connections with other neurons. These connections are shaped by genes and experience. During development, nerves connect by following chemical gradients that have been laid down by heredity. The connections are schematic, with lots of lines that later prove of little or no functional significance. Note that the connections are not fixed. Physical, sensory, and cognitive activity strengthen particular neural pathways, while those that are inactive fall by the wayside. Consequently, across generations the CNS has evolved by bits and pieces, guided by haphazard experience, not plan, and within the lifetime of an individual, the challenges of day-to-day life further refine the CNS connections established by evolution. The result is a mass of interconnected, overlapping neural networks that work in parallel and serial order. Each neuron, and there may be as many as 100 billion, is connected to thousands of other neurons, the neurons connect up in networks, and the neurons and networks change as a function of growth, physical activity, cognition, the demands of the environment, and all the various factors that influence psychological phenomena.

Neurons have three properties that are relevant to how drugs work and how the CNS works. They can maintain an electrical charge that differs from that of their immediate environment, they communicate by way of biochemical messages, and they are transformed by experience.

Neurons are excitable. They exist in one of two voltage-defined states, switching back and forth in milliseconds. One state registers a positive charge, the other registers a negative charge, and the difference is approximately 0.1 V. The two states and the transition from one to the other are mediated by charged biochemicals, called ions. The ions flow in and out of the neurons according to all the various events that influence psychological functioning, so that changes in voltage correspond to changes in psychological phenomena. These changes in voltage are analogous to the working of a light switch—on or off—or a computer chip—1 or 0. Consequently, there is a correspondence between psychological phenomena and the firing patterns of the billions of neurons that make up the nervous system. To take but one example, it is possible to see with your eyes closed, as in dreams, because the neural firing patterns mediate the relationship between reflected light and the experience of seeing. In other words, if the neural firing patterns are reinitiated, light is not needed.

Neurons send biochemical messages to each other, called neurotransmitters. The neurotransmitters are synthesized within the body of the neuron and then released upon prodding from other neurons or events in the environment. The neurotransmitters briefly hook up with neighboring neurons at subcellular sites called receptors. The receptor-bound neurotransmitters open up a channel in the recipient neuron, which then leads to a change in its firing pattern. For instance, vision comes about by photons setting off chemical reactions at the retina, which initiate the release of neurotransmitters, which in turn set off chains of electrical and biochemical activity in parallel networks of neurons. The result is visual experience. Similar chains of events occur with actions, emotions, ideas, and all else psychological.

Neurons are highly plastic. This plasticity subserves learning and all other experience-driven persistent changes in an individual. One of the major players in CNS plasticity is the receptor (the structure that receives chemical messages from other neurons). Experiments show that exercise, stress, sensory events, and thoughts modify the number of functional receptors and their affinity for different neurotransmitters. As our thoughts are mediated by the CNS and the CNS is plastic, our thoughts can modify the CNS and thereby modify future psychological functioning.

Drugs modify neurons and neuronal communication. On the basis of this background it is easy to see how drugs work. Neuronal excitability and neuron-to-neuron communication are mediated by chemicals. Drugs are chemicals. Thus drugs can alter neuron excitability and communication. Psychoactive drugs modify the CNS processes that subserve psychological phenomena. Some psychoactive drugs influence the synthesis of neurotransmitters, others mimic neurotransmitters, others influence the availability of neurotransmitters at the receptor sites, and so on. For example, heroin attaches to neurons that are involved in the mediation of pain and social stress. Cocaine promotes the functionality of dopamine, a neurotransmitter that mediates movement and motivation. These actions have a common end. They alter neuronal excitability and neurons' capacity to release and respond to neurotransmitters. Hence, psychoactive drugs alter perception, mood, awareness, and action.

Why a drug's psychological effects vary as a function of context. Implicit in this description of drug and brain interactions is that drugs do not directly modify psychological functions. Rather, they directly influence neurons. This brings us to a key observation. That a drug acts on neurons, or more specifically, acts on a subset of neurons, is why the cultural milieu, individual differences, and other contextual factors influence the response to the drug. Three factors lead to this conclusion.

First, given the simplicity of the neuron, psychological phenomena involve the activity of millions of neurons. Second, a particular drug directly influences a limited number of neurons—just those that have the "right" receptor. Third, given that psychological phenomena involve the workings of millions of different kinds of neurons, the drug-specific neurons are necessarily but one of many psychological influences. The billions of neurons that the drug does not bind to embody contextual and individual qualities, such as past experiences, cultural values, conventionality, respect for the law, and so on. Put broadly, these other neurons reflect variations in the setting and variations in the individual. Thus, the reaction to the drug depends on the unbound as well as the bound neurons, which is to say it depends on variations in the setting and the individual.

This account also helps make sense of why drugs are so attractive and also so toxic. Drug doses can be arbitrarily large, dwarfing the concentrations of their endogenous analogs (the neurotransmitters). This means that drugs can alter neurons in ways not matched by nondrug experiences. The consequences of arbitrarily large drug doses include tolerance, withdrawal, intoxication, the rush that attends heroin injections, and the various unique subjective experiences that drug users so often report. But intense subjective effects are on a continuum with toxicity, so that large doses of most psychoactive substances lead to tissue damage and are sometimes fatal.

That neurons mediate psychological phenomena helps make sense of the findings reported in this and later chapters. Historical trends, including shifts in values and attitudes, influence the likelihood that heroin use graduates to heroin addiction because psychological phenomena are embodied in the nervous system and heroin affects the nervous system. At the level of the CNS, values, ideas, expectations, and drugs take the same form (patterns of fluctuating action potentials) and are equally palpable.

3

ADDICTION IN THE FIRST PERSON

In this chapter drug users hold center stage. They—not researchers—describe drug use and addiction. Their stories establish a larger narrative—a natural history of drug use, constructed from the contributions of individual drug users. The first set of vignettes includes reports of the initial drug experiences, which were often quite positive. The next set of stories describes the tribulations of long-term drug use. These accounts include a mix of positive and negative experiences. The last set describes trying to quit drugs. These vignettes often have a surprising or ironic cast to them. Although addiction is not an ordinary occurrence, the reasons for quitting are often quite ordinary.

The biographical sketches fill a gap in the literature. Although the most salient feature of addictive drugs is their subjective effects, very little is published about this aspect of drug use. For example, the Web search terms "cocaine *and* subjective effects *and* human" returned twelve references, whereas the search terms "cocaine *and* dopamine" returned 1,846 references in *PsycINFO*, the primary internet behavioral science bibliographic service (July 24, 2008). Of course, the truthfulness of the biographical accounts is not guaranteed, and even if truthful, there is then the question of whether the accounts reveal a general truth or an idiosyncratic truth. Perhaps addicts who choose to talk about their experiences are more likely to have had bad experiences and feel a need to tell others, or, conversely, have not had such a bad time and are now in a position to tell their stories.

Researchers have evaluated the truthfulness of self-reports by checking what their informants say against biological assays that provide hard evidence of recent drug use. These studies are reviewed below. The question of whether the self-reports are representative of addiction is a more challenging question. It was dealt with by comparing the themes that emerged in the self-reports with the themes that emerged in the large, nationwide surveys introduced in the previous chapter. These surveys selected subjects that matched important U.S. demographic characteristics. Thus, if the two versions of addiction match up, we have strong evidence that the autobiographical accounts are not only true stories but are also representative stories of the inner life of addiction.

There is a straightforward way to check whether what people say about their drug use is true. The drugs and their residues, called metabolites, persist for some time in the circulatory system. For example, traces of heroin persist in the urine for hours, in blood for days, and in hair for months. Taking advantage of these facts, researchers have compared the biological data with verbal reports. The results are systematic and sensible. When the informant felt confident that a candid account would not result in punishment, then words told the same story as urine, blood, and hair samples. The correlations were typically above 0.75 (Darke, 1998; Weatherby et al., 1994). However, if the informants had reason to think that evidence of drug use might bring harm, they prudently denied any drug use (e.g., Land & Kushner, 1990; Nair et al., 1994; Ostrea et al., 1992). Thus, we can estimate the truthfulness of the stories that appear in this chapter by examining the circumstances under which they were obtained.

For the most part the interviews were carried out by researchers who did not have official ties with the judicial system or even clinics. In some cases the interviewers were from the same neighborhood as the subjects and were themselves once addicts. According to the research literature, these are the conditions that are most likely to promote honest reports. For instance, in a comprehensive review of the self-report literature, the correlations between the drug user's words and their tissue samples ranged from 0.58 to 1.0, with a median of 0.81 (Darke, 1998). The discrepancies were sometimes mistakes rather than deceit. For instance, someone would say that he or she had shot up two days ago, whereas the urine test indicated no drug use for at least three days. Shane Darke, an expert in this area of research, summarizes the findings in the following encouraging words:

> What is remarkable about the studies . . . is their consistency. Respectable reliability and validity has been obtained in the overwhelming majority of studies . . . The consistency of the findings of drug studies using different methodologies and in

different countries is further corroboration of the overall utility of self-report. Of course, if injecting drug users are asked questions in which truthful answers will result in negative consequences, valid responses should not be expected. (p. 262)

Thus, it is possible to obtain self-reports that are valid reflections of actual drug use.

Positive Initial Drug Experiences

Louis and Umber: Two inner city men comment on their first heroin experiences. The first two self-reports are from a monograph on Black male heroin users from East Coast, inner-city neighborhoods (Hanson, 1985). The authors state that their goal is "to learn more about the lifestyle(s) of hardcore, inner-city, Black male heroin users who had never been in treatment" (p. 189). The interviews lasted several hours, followed a common structure, and were conducted by former heroin addicts. The interviewees were long-term, current heroin users, whose lives revolved around their daily "fix." The unemployed addicts began their day with a scramble for money for their next high. These activities included conning money from friends and relatives, selling stolen goods, shoplifting, and various other minor scams. For those with the means, heroin was taken on schedule, once or twice a day. In short, the interviewees approximated the "street addict" or "junkie" stereotype.

> *Louis (18 years old at the time of the interview):* It started as a tingle in my toes and it went completely through my body, quickly through my head and I just relaxed as though I had taken a sedative. It just relaxed me and sorta gave me an upper . . . I found complete satisfaction . . . At first I felt exhilarated. Then it really started coming down and I just cooled out into my nod, and that was cool. It was cool. I hate to say that but it was. It was cool, man, that was it, there, buddy, the ultimate high. Fired up, brother. (p. 84)

> *Umber (26 years old at the time of the interview):* I felt a warm sensation over my whole body. My body relaxed, my hands relaxed, it felt like I had a shield up, ready for anything that come at me. It was a real good feeling. Made you feel like you didn't really need to care about nothing. (p. 84)

Louis and Umber had positive expectations. Their "cool" friends did heroin, and like their friends, they report a positive first experience.

Ann and Raffaella: Two women comment on initial use. Ann Marlowe is an Ivy League graduate; Raffaella Fletcher is from London. Marlowe inhaled powdered heroin nasally ("snorted") for about eight years (1999). In an article published in *Harvard Magazine,* she is described as a Harvard graduate, Columbia MBA, and "prosperous" headhunter for tax and pension attorneys (Lambert, 2000). Although often a regular heroin user and no stranger to withdrawal, she says that "I never felt it was a big deal. I could quit at any time, and I did."

> For a while nothing happened . . . And then came a surge of astonishing pleasure, in which I could think of nothing but how oddly benign the drug felt . . . It was like the best parts of a mushroom high, magnified ten times—euphoric, warm, comforting, and also controlled. No sloppy slack of being drunk. Everything was fine . . . it makes you feel everything is fine when it isn't. (pp. 23–24)

Raffaella Fletcher was attracted to drugs at an early age. At thirteen she began smoking marijuana and at eighteen turned to heroin. Like Marlowe, she had a talent for school work. But from her early teen years to early adulthood, drugs, not school, were her primary focus. Her autobiography, titled *Dangerous Candy* (1990), was co-written with Peter Mayle, the author of the best-selling *Year in Provence* (1991). In the next passage, Raffaella describes the first time she smoked marijuana. She is 13 years old and at a Rolling Stones concert. In the second passage, she describes the first time she tried heroin. She is now 18 years old and living with her boyfriend, having left home a few years earlier.

> There are plenty of people who don't like to accept a basic fact about drugs. They look at the end result and see misery or death . . . but they don't think about the beginning, that from the very first hit some drugs make some people feel fantastic . . . when it happens to you, you don't forget it. And you want more. Once is never enough.
>
> The joint and the beer and the music did it for me. I wasn't shy or awkward anymore. I was relaxed. I floated through the

evening. It wasn't a superhuman rush, but it was enough to make me feel that I understood what it was to get high. (pp. 8–9)

Raffaella Fletcher on her first heroin experience; her boyfriend injects her: He hit the vein, and within seconds the smack hit me. It came from my belly like cream and spread everywhere—warm, calm, dreamy, filling me up with a sensation that was like nothing I'd ever felt before. (pp. 22–23)

Silver: Feeling invincible and the most intense "nothingness." The following passage expands on Raffaella's comment that it "was like nothing I'd ever felt before." The author is 20 years old and calls himself "Silver." Unlike the first four narrators, Silver says he used heroin only once. The account can be found in the "Experiences Vault" of a Web site (*Erowid*, http://www.erowid.org) that invites submissions on mind-altering drugs, including self-reports of drug use.

Silver: Nothing could touch me. I was invincible, without the energy of being invincible. . . . the syringe is trying to make me feel bad . . . but it can't, nothing can. People always try to put into words the feeling smack brings you . . . that's just the problem . . . it doesn't . . . It was the most intense nothingness there ever was.

These informants lived in quite different environments: inner city, Ivy League schools, and London in the 1960s. Yet there are important similarities in their accounts of first use. The experiences were positive, unique, and included a sense of invulnerability. Umber volunteered that he felt like "he had a shield up," Ann felt like "everything was fine" when she knew that it wasn't, and Silver felt like he was beyond the reach of all threats: "nothing could touch me."

Miserable Initial Drug Experiences

Although the first five informants describe somewhat similar reactions, drug reactions are often quite different from person to person. For instance, a second theme in first-time heroin use is terrible nausea. This is because heroin acts on the brain's chemoreceptor area, sometimes called the "vomiting center." Heroin also inhibits brain areas that control breathing, with effects that can prove fatal. Both nausea and respiratory suppression abate with repeated use (tolerance) but do not disappear. These observations suggest that some people should respond quite negatively to opiates, particularly at first.

Dr. Ian Oswald: A week made utterly grim. In the next report, Dr. Ian Oswald, one of the pioneers of sleep research, describes what a week of heroin is like. In contrast to the first set of users, he was interested in withdrawal symptoms, not the initial rush. This rather strange pursuit was motivated by earlier observations that one of the symptoms of heroin withdrawal was highly disturbed sleep patterns. Oswald reasoned that by experiencing withdrawal himself, he might learn something about the biology of sleep. He served as his own guinea pig and managed to persuade a colleague to join him. He describes their experience as follows (cited in Latimer & Goldberg, 1981):

> We've been on heroin a week now . . . Seven days of voluntary illness. And how ill we feel . . . My personal view at present is just one made gray and utterly grim by heroin. The extraordinary thing is that it brings no joy, no pleasure. Weariness, above all. At most, some hours of disinterest—the world passing by while you feel untouched. Even after the injection there is no sort of thrill, no mind-expanding nonsense, no orgiastic heights, no Kubla Khan . . . You doze, see a daft scene where someone throws something, jump with a sort of panic, and doze again. Hypnagogic hallucinations, they're called . . . Why should people take this stuff—not for joy. Only for an hour of sudden shafts of panic and itching. (p. 7)

Manny Torres: From nausea to the perfect moment. A miserable first experience with a drug does not necessarily mean that it is not tried again. Manny Torres, introduced next, describes a horrible first experience, but then, under the influence of his friends and relatives, he gives it another try (Rettig et al., 1977).

> I close off one nostril, hold the other one and breathe in . . . My head start to spin, I start to throw up, and I say, "What the fuck did I do, Eddie?" Man . . . I was really sick; I felt terrible . . . "Man, I don't want no more of this. That's it, I've had it." (p. 33)

Eddie comes by the house. Manny is curious. If his uncle is always using heroin, it must be good:

> So I snort again and hey, it's really something else. I mean . . . you can't describe it. All the colors of Times Square tumble right over your forehead . . . like a million, jillion shooting stars . . .
>
> And the world levels out . . . There's no right, no wrong. Everything's beautiful, and it's like nothing's happening . . . but clear crisp light . . . And you want to gather all of creation inside you; maybe for a minute you do. What a perfect Manny Torres you become for a moment! (pp. 33–34)

These accounts of first experiences help explain the allure of heroin and other drugs. To say that heroin is "like nothing else" is to say that the experience has no clear likeness or precedent. If Raffaella wants to re-experience the feelings she had the first time she took heroin, she has only one choice: heroin. If Silver wants to feel "the most intense nothingness" once again, his only option is heroin. If Louis wants to feel both "cool" and "fired up," or if Ann wants to feel "oddly benign," their only choice is heroin. In contrast, the pleasures that come with other appetites can often be met by more than one substance or activity. Many different foods satisfy the pleasures of eating, many different physical activities satisfy the pleasures of movement, many different mental activities satisfy the pleasures of the mind. These observations say that part of the appeal of heroin, especially at first, is the uniqueness of its psychological effects. When it comes to "intense nothingness," heroin has the market cornered. Given that addictive drugs vary widely in terms of the receptors that they bind to and their pharmacological effects, they offer a wide range of unique subjective experiences.

Reflections on Addiction

The next set of informants describe regular drug use that has been in place for some time. Almost all are daily users of either heroin or cocaine, and their accounts make it clear that they would meet the *DSM* criteria for substance dependence. Their accounts vary. Some are bleak without respite. Others report great swings in mood, from the rigors of withdrawal to a fantastic high when they score some drug. Two informants voice no complaints and no regrets.

William S. Burroughs: The addict as a rabid dog. William S. Burroughs (1914–1997) led a long, eventful, and influential life. Along with Allen Ginsberg and Jack Kerouac he was among the best-known figures of the 1950s "Beat Generation." He wrote experimental fiction and evocative, hard-edged observations on drug use, using his own experience as his material. He is probably America's best-known opiate addict and certainly one of the most articulate. Recalling his years of opiate addiction while living in Tangier, Burroughs writes (1959):

> I lived in one room in the Native Quarter of Tangier. I had not
> taken a bath in a year nor changed my clothes or removed
> them except to stick a needle every hour in the fibrous grey
> wood flesh of terminal addiction . . . I could look at the end of
> my shoe for eight hours. I was only roused to action when the
> hourglass of junk ran out. If a friend came to visit—and they
> rarely did since who or what was left to visit—I sat there not car-
> ing that he had entered my field of vision—a grey screen always
> blanker and fainter—and not caring when he walked out of it.
> If he had died on the spot I would have sat there looking at my
> shoe waiting to go through his pockets. Wouldn't you? Because
> I never had enough junk—no one ever does. Thirty grains of
> morphine a day and it still was not enough. (p. xli)

There is no more vivid account of addiction as compulsion. According to Burroughs, the addict is "not in a position to act any other way":

> Junk yields a basic formula of "evil" virus: *The Algebra of Need*
> . . . A dope fiend is a man in total need of dope. Beyond a cer-
> tain frequency need knows absolutely no limit or control. In
> the words of total need: *"Wouldn't you?"* Yes you would. You
> would lie, cheat, inform on your friends, steal, do *anything* to
> satisfy total need. Because you would be in a state of total sick-
> ness, total possession, and not in a position to act in any other
> way. Dope fiends are sick people who cannot act other than
> they do. A rabid dog cannot choose but bite. (p. xxxix)

Manny Torres: "It anesthetizes the whole damn ugly world." The subtitle of Torres's autobiography is *A Criminal-Addict's Story* (Rettig et al., 1977). We learn that Manny grew up in a New York City neighborhood that was home to juvenile gangs, racketeers, and heroin. The book opens with Manny and his brother trying to score some heroin. For the last few days, they have been sleeping in parked cars to avoid the police. It is late at night and freezing outside.

> You're so damn sick . . . You're feeling so bad that you know you're going to die, and you have the remedy for all your problems right in your hand, That little dab of white powder is going to make you feel good . . .
>
> There is something fantastic and fatal about heroin, and no nonuser can ever dig it. Like it's the ultimate tranquilizer. It anesthetizes the whole damn ugly world. All your troubles become forgotten memories, lost on another dimension, when you're in the nod. And you don't even consider that it will soon wear off and the gentle nod will turn into a screaming want. And the nose-dripping, crawling, wormy feeling of needing a fix always follows the mellowest nod. (pp. 12–13)

Manny knows that heroin is what is making him sick, but he also knows that heroin is the quickest cure.

Frieda: An "addict who survived." The next vignette is from an oral history of drug use in America titled *Addicts Who Survived* (Courtwright et al., 1989). The respondents were veterans of America's first war against drugs. As the judicial implications of the Harrison Anti-Narcotic Act took hold, laws against illicit drug possession were more strictly enforced, federally funded drug research and rehabilitation hospitals were established, and the first Commissioner of the Federal Bureau of Narcotics successfully campaigned to include marijuana in the list of banned drugs. Many of those who remained regular heroin users did so behind the guise of legitimate jobs and otherwise conventional lifestyles. During the 1970s this population came to light. They were of special interest to researchers because their demographic ran against the street-addict stereotype. Little was known about older opiate addicts who worked nine to five.

Frieda is the oldest of the "addicts who survived." Like many in her cohort, she had avoided incarceration, and by her account was not involved in illegal activities other than opiate use. She started smoking opium in her early twenties. When opium became scarce and more expensive, she switched to heroin. When heroin supplies dried up during World War II, she took Dilaudid, a widely used opiate painkiller. In 1976, she lost her Dilaudid contact. Then, at age 77, she sought refuge in a methadone clinic. The interview takes place when Frieda is 81. She starts her story in the last year of the nineteenth century.

> I was born in 1899 in NYC . . . My parents were Jewish, but they were not religious people . . . I was the youngest of the six . . . I didn't graduate high school. I was just tired of school, that's all . . . I first started using drugs after I was divorced. I was smoking opium . . . All I felt was a good feeling. I kept going every night. I didn't think of the danger. I didn't think of nothing. I just smoked every night until I got hooked . . .
>
> When I couldn't get opium, I took heroin . . .
>
> I started to use Dilaudid. I lost my heroin connection on the Lower East Side. I got the Dilaudid from doctors. I got my needles from a druggist in the Bronx. He knew me for years. He must have known I was addicted . . .
>
> I entered the methadone program because I couldn't get Dilaudid . . .
>
> I want to stay on methadone. At my age, if I got off I'd die, I'd never make it.
>
> I'm happy. As long as I've got money and can play numbers, I'm happy. The whole day is spent playing numbers. I play numbers every day . . . I'm losing, losing, losing. I play a four, a five comes in; I play a five, a four comes in. But it keeps me going you know—something to do. (pp. 81–83)

In contrast to most of the other addicts, Frieda voices no regrets about years of drug use. She reports that she is satisfied with her life—as long as she can stay on methadone and bet on her numbers. According to the authors of *Addicts Who Survived*, all of the informants were asked if they "regretted" their years of opiate use. There is no direct reference to her answer to this question. However, she did volunteer that she was "happy."

Withdrawal

After extended use of an addictive drug, abstinence elicits a variety of physiological and psychological reactions, known as "withdrawal." These reactions reflect the compensatory biological changes that were induced by extended drug use. For example, the acute effects of opiates include sensations of warmth, muscular relaxation, constipation, elation, and sleepiness, whereas the withdrawal symptoms include chills, spasms, diarrhea, aches, depression, and restlessness. The best immediate cure for withdrawal symptoms is to start using the drug again. For instance, Manny Torres writes that he felt "so damn sick" but then, after shooting up, "[I] felt great . . . like a million dollars cash." The best long-term cure is to wait out the symptoms. Withdrawal symptoms dissipate in time, with the worst being over in a week or so.

Butch, Jim, Dap Daddy, and Ace: Inner-city men describe withdrawal. The excerpts are from the study on urban heroin addicts that included Louis and Usher, the first two informants in this chapter (Hanson, 1985). Butch is introduced first. His life is a mess. By his account this is largely a result of his deteriorating health and daily battle with withdrawal symptoms.

> *Butch:* My complexion is duller, I have a dull, hollow look. I don't seem as lively as other people. My dress is shabbier and it's getting shabbier and shabbier. I've had most of my teeth pulled . . . Heroin is something I have to take every day. When I don't get it I feel horrible. My hands are swollen . . . I become very impulsive. I get very angry over nonsense. You get in that drug slouch. You're so used to shooting heroin that you're nodding when you're not nodding . . . And if you're used to walking on a slouch when you're nodding, you're gonna walk that way when you ain't high. I was never born to be swollen like this. I wasn't born to limp, I wasn't born for my bowels to lock for me . . . You have that feeling about your swollen body, you don't want to really introduce yourself to nobody new because you're feeling that you're gonna be rejected. I have to be around where I can get my dope shot or I'm gonna be sick. (pp. 23–24)

> *Jim:* Rather than taking off, you feel deeply implanted. Rather than *going on a trip*, it [heroin] brings you back home. You don't go out like a jet or a rocket, you accommodate yourself to this world. (p. 89)

> *Dap Daddy:* It's my relaxer, *my shot* for the day . . . so I can feel *normal*. (p. 90)

Ace: Getting high is the *norm* for me . . . I just get *normal.*
(p. 90)

For Ace, Dap Daddy, Jim, and Butch heroin has lost much of its luster. It no longer produces indescribable highs. It "cures" some of the residual, negative long-term effects, but only for a while. On balance things are worse than before heroin use began.

Nancy: Managing long-term drug use. Nancy is a long-term, daily cocaine user. She did a few lines every day while keeping up with work, chores at home, and even visits to the gym. Her story is one of many found in an interesting study of San Francisco Bay Area cocaine addicts (Waldorf et al., 1991). The sample is unusual as measured by the standards of drug research. Most of the subjects had gone to college, were employed, were married, and worked in professions such as law and social work. Very few had been in jail or dealt drugs. By demographic criteria they are representative of the larger Bay Area population, but not of the addicts who typically populate research studies. According to Dan Waldorf and his colleagues who ran the study, Nancy is one of cocaine's "silent majority."

> Nancy is a very dynamic, well-organized woman who seems to have it all—a challenging career, a good marriage . . . healthy children, a nice home, money in the bank, and a secure future . . . Between 1974 and 1980 she used cocaine intermittently at parties or when her husband purchased some from time to time. On one occasion she injected the drug . . .
>
> Her cocaine use began to escalate when a close friend and colleague, Eva, began to sell cocaine to a small network of friends. The general pattern of her use was as follows: She arrived at work at eight o'clock, and did her most demanding creative work before noon. She then went to a gym for her regular workout and had lunch at one. Upon returning to the office she worked for another hour or so and then she and Eva would "do a line." At that point she put aside her creative work and dealt with the general administrative aspects of her job. At four or four-thirty she often had another line, and another at six just before she left work.
>
> Upon arriving home she generally had a drink and then pre-

pared the evening meal for her husband and their children. Sometimes just before eating, she would go to the bathroom and take a fourth line . . . After dinner she and her husband would clean up the dishes, put the kids to bed, rest or read for a while and then go to bed about 10:30 or 11:00 P.M. (pp. 144–145)

For a few years this pattern alternated with periods of even heavier use that also included a few extra lines of cocaine at night at a local bar. But, according to Nancy, there were no interruptions at work. Following the birth of her third child, she markedly decreased her cocaine intake (with no explanation why), and then (except on "special occasions") stopped for good.

There is not one theme that captures all of the reports. Some informants have nothing positive to say about their lives. On the other hand, Frieda and Nancy volunteered no complaints. However, if asked, I think most would have said that on balance they were better off before they became heavy drug users. For example, even Nancy quit using cocaine, something she would not have done if daily lines of cocaine really did make life better on balance. But the focus on overall benefits misses an important observation. For a short time the drugs provided significant relief. For a moment, Manny was "a perfect Manny Torres," and Butch stopped feeling so miserably "swelled up" and "sick."

On Quitting

Addiction is typically described as a "chronic, relapsing disease." The words "chronic, relapsing" imply that most addicts try to quit and in fact do remain abstinent for a while but then return to heavy drug use. In support of this point, the biographical literature includes many accounts of trying to quit.

The first case is from a monograph titled *Pathways from Heroin Addiction*. The author, Patrick Biernacki, interviewed 101 men and women who had been addicts but then quit without professional help, a process that is sometimes referred to as "natural" or "unassisted" recovery. The average number of years of heavy use was about six, and they had typically quit when they were about 27 years old (Biernacki, 1986). At the time of the research, the average number of years since the end of heavy drug use was also about six years.

In the preface, Biernacki explains that in focusing on "natural recovery" he is not suggesting that it is safe to experiment with heroin or that he is belittling the often devastating effects of heroin. Rather, his aim is to draw attention to a population of addicts that are typically not studied. Biernacki begins his book with a case study of a daily heroin user, a man he calls "Scott."

Scott: When the weekly salary is no longer sufficient. At the time of the study Scott was 42 years old and married for a second time. He describes his childhood and adolescence as happy, normal, comfortable, and middle class. Like many of his peers, he experimented with alcohol and marijuana in high school and college, but was otherwise a law-abiding young man. At age 21 he tried heroin for the first time and recalls that he "liked it right off." The following passage describes Biernacki's history of Scott's heroin addiction.

> For about four years Scott was addicted to heroin (e.g., a daily user). His marriage dissolved, but he managed to keep his job. He had a stable drug source, and aside from when he purchased the drug, he did not associate with other addicts, distancing himself from the street-addict scene.
>
> Heroin was expensive. When his salary could no longer support his habit, he borrowed money from his bank and credit union. Once he cashed stolen payroll checks to buy heroin, but this, reports Scott, was out of character. Although Scott was employed full time, heroin eventually drained all of his financial resources, including his credit line. As Scott puts it, he "had gone as far as [he] could go." He relays the following history of what he thought at the time:
>
> "[T]he only way [I] was going to be able to manage it was to start dealing drugs, and [I] didn't want to take the chance of getting busted. And second of all, to deal I'd have to be available all the time at strange hours. I couldn't have people call me up at work to score . . . It finally became clear that this was the end. I was going to have to make a big change, of my whole life . . . So that's why it was kind of a rational decision." (pp. 1–8, 52)

Scott shut himself up in a hotel room and withdrew from heroin. Scott had been a heroin addict for four years (on a daily basis), a methamphetamine addict for a year and a half (on a daily basis), and a frequent user of marijuana and LSD. At the time of the interview, Scott had not used heroin for more than ten years, had remarried, and was employed.

The next three informants were subjects in the San Francisco Bay Area cocaine study that included Nancy, previously described in this chapter. Recall that their demographic characteristics approximated those of the general population of San Francisco. The subjects were typically well educated and employed (Waldorf et al., 1991). Harry, whose story best fits common understandings of addiction, is presented first.

Harry: Ruins career and marriage, then quits cocaine. Harry is described as an active, successful, and highly social young man. Prior to becoming a heavy cocaine user, he was a stockbroker by day and law student at night. In between work and school he pursued a busy social life that included regular but not heavy use of cocaine, mostly on the weekends (perhaps 1 gram a week on average). After passing the bar Harry started a private practice. It was, he reports, an immediate success. At about the same time he began using more cocaine and switched modes of self-administration. He started smoking cocaine (called freebasing), a process that produces a more powerful high than nasal self-administration. To keep his growing habit a secret from his wife and family, he rented an apartment to be used just for freebasing. Shielded from scrutiny, his intake shot up further to 28 grams a week (about an ounce) and then to more than 50 grams a week. All in all, his transition from law student to successful lawyer was accompanied by about a fifty-fold increase in weekly cocaine consumption.

Even for a successful lawyer, this much cocaine was a serious financial strain (about $5,000/week). Harry began to embezzle money from his clients to pay for his drugs. Following a car accident, which he attributed to lack of sleep, he made his first of several attempts to quit cocaine. The last attempt took place in an inpatient cocaine treatment center. Upon release, he became a regular attendee at Cocaine Anonymous and has since remained free of cocaine.

Harry says he has become "a more insightful, spiritual, and calm person, but it hasn't been easy." His wife divorced him, and he changed professions. Instead of law, he was working as a counselor in a drug and alcohol treatment program and attending psychology courses in preparation for graduate study. The authors report that he hopes to become a therapist.

Harry's story is noteworthy in that it so closely approximates the popular image of the cocaine addict—except for the last part about quitting. He lost his wife and career to cocaine. He embezzled money from his clients. He rented a second residence so that he could freebase without his family knowing what he was doing. Yet he did quit. Based on the dates provided in the ethnography, his drug career was about five to six years long, including two years of light use while in law school. From about the ages of 28 to 32, Harry fit the criteria of a "relapsing, chronic cocaine addict." At age 33, he no longer did.

There is no way to check if Harry really did quit and for how long. However, we can check something much more important. Is Harry's story typical? Taken literally, his story predicts that most heavy cocaine users will quit by their early thirties. Indeed, given that Harry became a heavy cocaine user later in life than is usual, if Harry's story is typical, then most heavy cocaine users will have quit by the end of their twenties. This is tested in the next chapter.

Jessie: Unassisted quitting and learning to ignore cocaine cravings. Jessie was 28 years old at the time of his interview. His story starts when he switched from snorting cocaine to smoking cocaine. As did Harry, he liked freebasing because the high came on so quickly and powerfully, and like Harry, once he started freebasing, his cocaine consumption began to accelerate. In a short while he was using every day and while on the job, something he had not done before. Jessie estimates that during his peak period, he was consuming about six grams of cocaine a week.

With heavy use came heavy costs. Jessie was spending more than $500/ week on drugs. This was well beyond his means. He started falling behind on his bills, not doing well at work, and losing weight. As he put it, his life had "gone out of control." To stem the losses and regain control, he concluded that he would have to quit cocaine. He says:

> At first it's like you hit the pipe and then go home. But then it got to be that we were doing this every night, and I started doing it on our lunch hour. (p. 127)
> It went on for months on almost an everyday basis . . . I was

actually getting high all the time. I could even sit at home and actually taste it. Then you start making excuses why you should. It just progressed and then I just stopped paying bills and the shit started going down the tubes . . . Between the drug and the pressures of not taking care of your responsibilities . . . my brain was about to just bomb. I just had to stop. I remember the night I stopped . . . I had done a gram. When I get high I start thinking and I decided I couldn't do it anymore. That night I made up my mind to not do it and I didn't. The next day I said to them, "Don't come out with it," and they respected that. (p. 128)

After following through on his vow to quit, Jessie was tempted to use again. He experienced cravings for cocaine. Friends, drug paraphernalia, even thoughts of cocaine triggered the desire to take it—just as thoughts of a loved one inspire longing. Jessie describes his response to cocaine cravings in the following words:

You can sit there and you can taste it or you could be sitting there and all of a sudden just smell it. Then you start thinkin' about it. I just had to keep telling myself, "No, you can't do this." (p. 129)

After a while his cravings faded.

Patty: Cocaine or food on the table? Patty is a single mother of two girls and for fifteen years was a heavy cocaine user (Waldorf et al., 1991). To maintain her family and also keep herself in cocaine, she sold drugs and worked in a bank. Dealing is risky, and one day Patty was almost arrested. The close call convinced her to quit selling drugs. But without the extra income, she faced a dilemma: food on the table for her girls or cocaine. She describes her thought processes in the following terms:

Yeah, the girls were getting older and starting to have friends over, and it started getting embarrassing, because people are coming to pick up something and other kids are there and my kids are embarrassed. I'm also a P.T.A. president, right, and that is going to look fuckin' great when I get busted . . . (p. 200)

Oh, for a time my nose opened up when I went out partying and drinking, but I learned how to handle it. You know, I never really decided to quit using. I just quit selling. Once I stopped selling I didn't have the money to buy it anymore. I would have literally had to say, "Sorry, girls, you don't eat this week" to buy some. I would have exactly $80 for two weeks of food. (p. 202)

Patty is concerned about the material and psychological welfare of her girls and also their regard for her. She worries that she might embarrass her daughters, and this concern, although conjectural, dominates her present and palpable cocaine cravings. For example, she recalls that situations that were associated with snorting cocaine elicited cravings, but like Jessie, she implies that she learned to ignore them: "Oh, for a time my nose opened up when I went out partying and drinking."

QUITTING HEROIN

The next section identifies three different endings to heavy heroin use. Their common feature is that unlike for Scott, who started this section, heroin use does not stop all at once. The first narrative is about a young woman who cuts down from three injections of heroin a day to about one a week. She became a controlled heroin user, referred to on the street and in the research literature as a "chipper." Her story is told by the late Dr. Norman Zinberg and his colleagues (1977). Zinberg is often referred to as a pioneer of addiction research and was particularly interested in the factors that allowed for the controlled use of addictive drugs.

Linda: From heavy user to chipper. Linda started using marijuana in high school. She reports being "infatuated" with the marijuana high, but remained a social, weekend smoker. In college she dealt marijuana to her friends for "kicks" and "excitement." She did well in school but quit after her first year and hitchhiked to California. She said she hoped to become a "junkie." She added that she had no idea what that meant, except that she had heard that "junk" was the best high in the world. In California she started shooting heroin and was soon up to three injections a day. Following the arrest of her boyfriend she returned to the East Coast. She cut back on heroin and then stopped completely when she became pregnant. After her child was born, she began using again, but not daily. The article reports that for six years she has been smoking—and occasionally injecting—heroin with friends on about a weekly basis. Linda says that she does not share needles and arranges her heroin days so that getting high does not interfere with her job or taking care of her child.

Zinberg explained heroin chipping in terms that apply to social drinking. Chippers developed rituals and practices that protected their conventional lives from their weekend heroin bouts. For instance, they put aside a fixed amount of drug and disapproved of anyone who exceeded their preset ration. It is likely that Zinberg's heroin chippers also differed in other ways from the heroin addicts who usually participate in research studies. For instance, Zinberg's account suggested that they were more likely to be employed and were more highly educated. This and related questions have not been pursued any further. However, what is certain is that chipping is a general phenomenon, found with all addictive drugs. Indeed, a good proportion of the current U.S. population are "alcohol chippers."

Wendy: Moral qualms and drifting into abstinence. Wendy is a mother and an ex–heroin addict. She dates the beginning of her exit from heroin addiction to a transformative experience. One of the primary features of this experience was the realization that she wanted her parents and her son to be proud of her (cited in Jorquez, 1983).

> One evening (while in the California desert) I climbed on this big rock, and just sat there alone waiting for the sunset. It was beautiful. Then I snapped . . . "What am I doing? God did not put me here on this earth to be using heroin!" For the first time I felt guilty about being a user. I began to have these powerful feelings for my parents to be proud of me again. And I thought about my son and my responsibilities to him. I stayed clean for about two weeks that time. (p. 353)

Wendy's stated motivations for quitting are similar to Patty's: family relations were in conflict with drug use. However, according to the article in which this account appears, Wendy used for several more years, then gradually "drifted" into abstinence. This slow transition stands in contrast to the cold-turkey approaches of Scott, Jessie, and Patty, and it also suggests that feelings of guilt were not the only reasons she eventually quit using heroin.

Words and deeds: Did morphine really trump all other motivations for William Burroughs? Recall that William Burroughs, who introduced the section on long-term heavy use, explained that he, like other opiate addicts, couldn't do otherwise because he "never had enough junk." But Patty, Jessie, and Scott quit. They said they did so for economic reasons and in Patty's case concern for family. Burroughs, on the other hand, was shielded from economic concerns. Although more than 40 years old, Burroughs was living off a stipend from his family (Morgan, 1988). He was not self-supporting; he had an allowance. But then for reasons that his biographer did not specify, the checks from home stopped coming. Without his allowance, Burroughs came up against the same dilemma that Scott, Patty, and Jessie faced: somehow get more money, perhaps by dealing drugs, or quit. Burroughs had heard of a London clinic that had developed a new experimental treatment for heroin addiction. He writes, referring back to the same period of time that he was at the height of his opiate addiction (1959): "I stood there with my last check in my hand and realized that it was my last check. I took the next plane to London" (p. xlii).

Burroughs says his London cure involved sessions of apomorphine, forced vomiting, and abstinence. It is a curious story. Apomorphine does not bind to opiate receptors, and it is not a known treatment for opiate addiction. Nevertheless, Burroughs lived the rest of his life as a productive writer and culture icon. According to his friends, he continued to use opiates from time to time, but, apparently like Linda, not in a way that interfered with his other interests.

No one describes drug craving and compulsive drug use as vividly as does Burroughs (a wooden arm, made fibrous by the morphine needle). Yet as soon as the checks from home stopped arriving, he decided to do otherwise.

Not Quitting

Not all addicts quit using. Some of the narrators in this chapter said nothing about quitting, although many focused on the penalties of regular heroin and cocaine. The next and last narrative is that of someone who also gives no sign of quitting. The story is told by Dr. Avram Goldstein (1994). Goldstein was an early champion of methadone, a pharmacological treatment for heroin, and an early and influential opiate psychopharmacologist. He begins his book with the story of a heroin addict who has just been released from jail. Goldstein's point is that this is someone who should quit using heroin but doesn't:

> A 50-year-old man gets off the bus in a seedy downtown neighborhood. Just hours before, he was released after serving a two-year sentence for burglary, his third time in prison. His regular income as a grocery clerk had barely been enough to support his wife and child, so burglary seemed the only way to raise the large sums he needed for his heroin habit. Watch him! Only a block from the bus terminal, he makes his "connection," buys a syringe and needle and some white powder. Heroin put him in prison three times, heroin will surely finish him off. Why doesn't he quit? Why didn't he quit 25 years ago, when he could see clearly enough what his future would be if he continued using heroin? (p. 1)

The stories in this chapter tell a cautionary tale. At first the drug experiences were indescribably great. The informants said that they were swept away by feelings of connectedness, tranquility, and competence: "cool and fired up," "ready for anything," "best parts of a mushroom high, magnified ten times," "controlled, no sloppy slack of being drunk," "nothing could touch me . . . I was invincible without the energy of being invincible." But as drug consumption continued, the ecstasy faded and was replaced by withdrawal symptoms, health problems, career problems, and financial problems. Some informants openly acknowledged that drug use was the source of their difficulties, yet they kept using the drugs. Others quit. Those who discussed their motives for quitting often mentioned financial concerns and indicated that they would have to start selling drugs to make ends meet. William Burroughs quit, at least temporarily, when his allowance from home stopped showing up. Two informants, Patty and Wendy, explained quitting in terms of family obligations and a desire to avoid family conflict.

When addicts speak for themselves, quitting drugs becomes part of the story of addiction. This is a provocative finding. It suggests that the claim that addiction is a chronic disease may not be true. Indeed, the autobiographies suggest that most addicts will be ex-addicts by the time they are 30 years old. In the next chapter this hypothesis is put to the test.

4

ONCE AN ADDICT, ALWAYS AN ADDICT?

The prognosis for addiction is bleak. According to most clinicians and researchers, an addict is someone for whom sobriety is a tenuous and temporary state; addicts almost always resume drug use, even if free of drugs for years. For instance, Charles P. O'Brien and A. Thomas McLellan, two widely published addiction researchers, note that most addicts relapse, that "cure" is an unrealistic hope, and that "[a]ddictive disorders should be considered in the category with other disorders that require long-term or lifelong treatment" (1996, p. 239; McLellan et al., 2000). They group addiction with other long-term conditions such as arthritis, asthma, and diabetes. In an article published in *Science*, Alan Leshner (1997), director of NIDA during the "decade of the brain," added Alzheimer's and schizophrenia to the list of disorders resembling addiction. Treatment organizations, such as Alcoholics Anonymous and Narcotics Anonymous, and psychiatric textbooks refer to abstinent addicts as "recovering," not "recovered," regardless of how long they have been off drugs. Summarizing these views, the authors of the chapter on substance use disorders in the *Textbook of Clinical Psychiatry* write: "For addiction patients, recovery is a never-ending process; the term *cure* is avoided." (Mack et al., 2003, p. 341). Presaging current expert opinion, Charles Dederich, the founder of Synanon, a residential treatment program for heroin addicts that came to prominence in the 1960s, states: "We once had the idea of graduates . . . This was a sop to social workers and professionals . . . A person with this fatal disease will have to live here all his life" (cited in Brecher, 1972). Dederich no longer needs to hide the "facts." The expression "once an addict, always an addict" has become the mainstream view.

This gloomy vision of the addict's prospects is not without empirical support. Some research does show that those who enter treatment for addiction never really stop using drugs or resume use shortly after treatment ends. A chapter in an old but an excellent book, *Licit and Illicit Drugs* (Brecher, 1972), includes a review of the major approaches to opiate treatment for the first half-century of American anti-drug programs. The techniques included sanitariums, detoxification centers, and community-oriented residential treatment centers. None worked. About 80 to 90 percent of the patients resumed drug use within a year or so after the end of the program. Brecher writes:

> No effective cure for heroin addiction has been found—neither rapid withdrawal, nor gradual withdrawal, neither the drug sanitariums . . . nor long terms of imprisonment . . . nor Lexington . . . nor the California program . . . nor the New York State program . . . nor the National Addiction Rehabilitation Administration program . . . nor Synanon . . . nor the other therapeutic communities. Nor should this uninterrupted series of failures surprise us. *For heroin really is an addicting drug.* (p. 83)

This was written in 1972. Thirty-three years later, prominent addiction researcher A. Thomas McLellan and his colleagues offer an update (2005). They contend that for all drugs of abuse, not just heroin, relapse is the expected treatment outcome:

> In fact, most alcohol- and drug-dependent patients relapse following cessation of treatment . . . In general about 50–60% of patients begin re-using within six months following treatment cessation, regardless of the type of discharge, the patient characteristics or the particular substance(s) of abuse. (p. 449)

Clinic studies are also spotlighted in psychiatric texts. In the *Sourcebook on Substance Abuse*, the chapter titled "Relapse Prevention" starts with the sentence (Ott et al., 1999): "Outcome studies show that the majority of individuals who receive treatment for substance use disorders relapse." Thus, the claim that addiction is a chronic relapsing disorder can be backed up by more than a hundred years of research. Clinical records show that addicts who enter treatment often relapse.

When addicts speak for themselves, the story turns to quitting, however. Many of the heavy drug users featured in the last chapter quit. Scott was a daily methamphetamine user, then a daily heroin user; Jessie was doing cocaine at work and at home, and Patty used cocaine for fifteen years. Yet they quit. A common theme was that quitting came about as the responsibilities of adulthood took on greater importance. Recall that Jessie was worried about his utility bills, Scott was worried he would lose his job, and Patty was worried about groceries. If we drew a graph of these stories, putting age on the horizontal axis and drug use on the vertical axis, the curve would peak in the mid-twenties and then rapidly decline. This is a rather different picture than that portrayed in the clinical texts, the pages of *Lancet* and the *Journal of the American Medical Association.*

Who Is Right?

The addicts of the last chapter and the experts presented in this chapter disagree. Who is right? Unfortunately, on the basis of the facts that each group provides, it is not possible to tell. Self-reports are subject to various distortions, and even if valid may reflect the exceptions rather than the rule. The clinical texts and expert opinions just cited are also based on life histories that may not be representative of the typical life history. Addiction researchers have relied largely on addicts who are in treatment, but most of those who meet the criteria for addiction were never in treatment. In one of the largest national surveys of psychiatric health and treatment, the Epidemiologic Catchment Area study, just 30 percent of those who met the criteria for dependence or abuse had ever brought their drug problems to the attention of a health specialist (Anthony & Helzer, 1991). Note that the criterion was not treatment, but simply saying "yes" to the question, "did you mention your drug use to a health specialist?" In a follow-up national survey conducted in 2001–2002 that recruited more than 43,000 subjects for face-to-face interviews, 16 percent of those who met the criteria for substance dependence were in treatment (Stinson et al., 2005). In this survey, treatment was broadly, albeit more precisely, defined. It included religious counseling, self-help groups, outpatient care, inpatient detoxification, and eleven other distinct forms. Thus, the factual basis for the claim that addiction is a chronic, relapsing disorder is based on populations that also may be unrepresentative of addicts as a whole.

Indeed, the clinic populations that provide the factual basis for the claim that addiction is a chronic, relapsing, lifelong disorder are by definition not representative: they were in treatment. Of course this does not, in itself, mean that they are unrepresentative of the natural history of addiction; it may typically persist for years and years so that Scott and the others introduced in the last chapter are outliers. But a well-known bias in medical research, called "Berkson's bias," suggests that addicts in treatment may be the least likely to stop using drugs. Berkson's bias refers to the fact that patients who are in treatment for a particular disorder are more likely to suffer from additional disorders that are independent of the disease in question (Berkson, 1946; Maric et al., 2004). Consequently the course of the disease is more serious, but this is exogenous, due to interactions with the additional symptoms. Thus, if addicts with additional disorders are the ones who end up in the clinic, and if these disorders increase the likelihood of relapse, addicts in clinics will be the least likely to stop using. What is needed are studies that select heavy drug users independent of whether or not they are in treatment.

How to Test Whether Addiction Is a Chronic Disorder

There are straightforward ways to determine whether addiction is usually a chronic disorder. One has to do with when heavy drug use starts; the other involves the average age of the samples in the epidemiological studies. Most of those who become addicts typically start using drugs heavily in their late teens or early twenties. In surveys that select subjects at random who are at least 18 years old, the median age is more than 40 (nationalatlas.gov). If "chronic" means at least ten years of heavy drug use, so that addiction typically persists well past age 30, then most of those who ever met the criteria for dependence would still do so at the time that the survey was conducted. However, if drug use in addicts typically declines to subclinical levels after five years or so, then most lifetime addicts will be ex-addicts at the time of the survey. For example, if the likelihood of addiction coming to a halt in any given year averaged about 25 percent, then the likelihood of addiction lasting more than five years would be less than 70 percent. In this example, most cases of addiction would be resolved by about age 28 or so, which is younger than the median age for the study population.

To properly carry out this test, it is essential to recruit a large number of subjects. For instance, if lifetime addiction rates were 5 percent, then it would be necessary to recruit 20,000 subjects to insure approximately 1,000 lifetime addicts. The studies reported next followed this strategy.

But before reviewing the data, a qualification is in order regarding what is being tested. The phrase "addiction is a chronic, relapsing disease" entails three separable claims. In this chapter the research results test whether or not addiction is chronic. This is understood to mean that addicts typically use for ten or more years so that they still meet the criteria for dependence when they are well into their thirties, and that addiction lasts at least as long as the average psychiatric disorder. During the active phase of heavy drug use, say when the user is in his twenties, the pattern may be relapsing in the sense that periods of heavy use are punctuated by relatively brief periods of controlled use or abstinence.

Remission Rates in Large National Surveys

There are four large national studies that recruited representative populations and provide data relevant to relapse and remission rates for addiction (Anthony & Helzer, 1991; Kessler et al., 2005a, 2005b; Stinson et al., 2005, 2006; Warner et al., 1995). Although these studies were conducted by leading researchers and funded by various national health institutes, the findings have not become a staple of discussions of the nature of addiction. For example, none of the clinical texts and journal articles cited in the introduction to this chapter reference these epidemiological studies. Thus, one of the goals of this chapter—and this book—is to introduce this information to addiction researchers as well as the public, although the research itself is not new.

The Epidemiologic Catchment Area Study (1980–1984). The Epidemiologic Catchment Area (ECA) Study was the first nationwide epidemiological study to use the American Psychiatric Association's revised criteria for identifying cases. The revisions were motivated by the failure of earlier diagnostic criteria to provide reliable diagnoses. As its sponsors hoped, the changes markedly improved agreement among clinicians and researchers (Spitzer & Fleiss, 1974; Spitzer & Forman, 1979; Spitzer et al., 1979; Spitzer et al., 1980). The importance of this cannot be overestimated. Science requires the ability to check the findings of other researchers. Thus, if there are no agreed-upon rules for identifying who is an addict, a science of addiction is not possible.

The ECA study got off the ground in 1980 and took four years to complete. Subjects were recruited from five major metropolitan regions. Each region had its own research staff so that the findings from one region could be checked against those of the other four. This helped to prevent any markedly aberrant results. In each region, subjects were selected so as to produce a sample that was representative of the nation as a whole. The catchment areas included households, prisons, psychiatric hospitals, and nursing homes. Groups known to be more at risk, such as prisoners, were oversampled so as to insure reliable estimates of low-occurring disorders. Treatment was not a criterion. The data were then mathematically adjusted so that the overall prevalence rates would provide an accurate picture of the psychiatric health of the nation. In the end more than 19,000 subjects participated. In a foreword, Daniel X. Freedman, longtime editor of the *Archives of American Psychiatry* and a leading spokesman for science-based clinical practice, wrote (1991), "Here then is the soundest fundamental information about the range, extent and variety of psychiatric disorders ever assembled. In psychiatry, no single volume of the twentieth century has such importance and utility not just for the present but for the decades ahead" (p. xxiv).

Freedman's words are important. If the data are, as he says, the "soundest fundamental information" available on the "extent of psychiatric disorders," then they promise to answer the question of whether addiction is typically a chronic disorder.

Remission rates in the ECA survey. The next figure summarizes the ECA findings on remission. It shows the percentage of individuals who reported no drug-related problems for at least twelve months prior to the survey, but had met the lifetime criteria for drug dependence or drug abuse (based on Table 6.22 in Anthony & Helzer, 1991). The data are organized in terms of gender and age. For example, according to the biographies, remission rates should top 50 percent by age 30.

Figure 4.1 shows that at approximately age 24 more than half of those who ever met the criteria for addiction no longer reported even one symptom, and that by about age 37 approximately 75 percent of those who ever met the criteria for dependence were no longer reporting any symptoms. Since dependence requires at least three symptoms over a twelve-month period, it is likely that the proportion of those in their thirties who were still dependent was actually less than 25 percent. Also note that it must be the case that most of those who quit did so outside of the purview of drug treatment clinics. This follows from the facts that the most recent large psychiatric survey reported that only about 16 percent of those who were dependent were also in treatment, and that in the ECA survey approximately 30 percent of those who met the lifetime criteria for drug abuse and dependence had ever mentioned a drug prob-

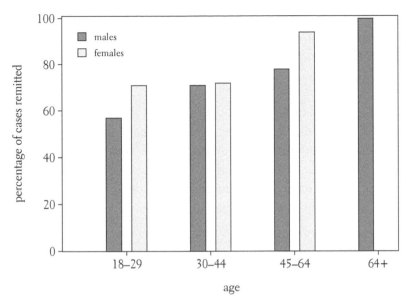

4.1 Remission for drug abuse and dependence as a function of age and gender in the ECA survey. Data are from Table 6.22 in Anthony and Helzer, 1991.

lem to a health specialist. These findings do not support the view that addiction is a chronic disease.

The National Comorbidity Survey (NCS), 1990–92 and replication (2001–02). If this last figure correctly reflects the natural history of addiction, then other studies that recruit representative samples should produce similar results. At the moment there are three such surveys plus a few smaller ethnographic studies. These will be reviewed, with some emphasis on methods so that we can insure that the high recovery rates were not a quirk of the ECA methods.

In the early 1990s and then again in the years 2001–2002, Ronald Kessler directed two large, nationwide surveys of mental health and mental health services (Kessler et al., 2005a, 2005b; Warner et al., 1995). As was the case with the ECA study, the goal was to provide an unbiased scientific account of key characteristics of psychiatric disorders. The research reports emphasized the associations between different disorders (e.g., the correlation between depression and addiction), and hence the project was titled the National Comorbidity Survey. In addition to comorbidity, the measures included lifetime prevalence rates, current prevalence rates, age of onset, and demographic indices. But, in contrast to the ECA survey, nonmetropolitan as well as metropolitan areas were sampled. There were about 8,100 and 9,300 subjects in the two NCS studies.

Figure 4.2 compares the remission rates for the ECA and 1990–1992 National Comorbidity surveys. Not counting addiction, the two surveys were in close agreement. The average (absolute) difference in remission rates was just 4 percent. For addiction, however, the two surveys came up with very different estimates of the percentage of "ex-addicts." The NCS reported that 74 percent of lifetime addicts were in remission, an even

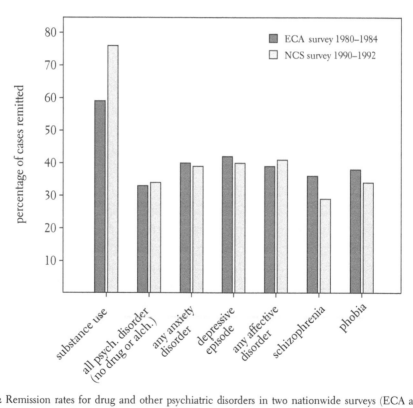

4.2 Remission rates for drug and other psychiatric disorders in two nationwide surveys (ECA and NCS). Remission for drug dependence (NCS) is about twice as high as for other psychiatric disorders. ECA remission rates are from Tables 4.3 and 13.8 of Robins & Regier, 1991; also Regier et al., 1990 and Table 6.22 in Anthony and Helzer, 1991. NCS remission rates are from data in Kessler et al., 1994, and Warner et al., 1995.

higher rate than the ECA study (59 percent). This is by far the largest difference between the two studies.[1]

The difference is due to two factors. First, the ECA survey used a much more liberal standard for counting current cases. Instead of the typical three symptoms, only one symptom was needed. In support of this point, when the NCS researchers recalculated their current addiction rates, remission rates decreased (from 74 to 63 percent) toward the ECA result. Second, the ECA mixed together abuse and dependence cases, and the typical finding is that abuse persists longer than does dependence (e.g., Vaillant, 1995). Thus, the differences in the ECA and NCS results are exactly what is expected given the different methods. Put another way, the differences are confirmation that the methods were reliable.

Double-checking the high remission rates. Since 1992, there have been two more large national studies of the prevalence of psychiatric disorders. Between 2001 and 2002, Kessler and his colleagues reran their study of drug dependence and its psychiatric correlates. At about the same time, the National Institute on Alcohol Abuse and Alcoholism sponsored the largest survey yet of substance disorders and their correlates (e.g., Grant & Dawson, 2006; Stinson et al., 2005, 2006). The NIAAA survey was motivated by many of the same goals as the ECA and NCS surveys, but their subject pool was larger—more than 43,000 subjects—and they appear to have gathered more detailed information on the psychiatric correlates of drug use. Figure 4.3 summarizes the results from all four surveys, with the data arranged chronologically to check for a historical trend.

The results are similar to the earlier results. Indeed the remission rates are slightly higher than reported in the first NCS study. Although the surveys were carried out in three different decades—the eighties, nineties, and aughts—with different populations, in different geographic regions of the country, and by different interviewers, they converge on the same result. Most individuals who met the criteria for lifetime addiction were no longer addicted at the time of the survey. Given the median age of the subject populations and the data presented in Figure 4.1, it is highly likely that most stopped using drugs at clinically significant levels in their late twenties or early thirties. High remission rates are a stable feature of addiction.

The claim that addiction is a chronic disorder is one of the staples of

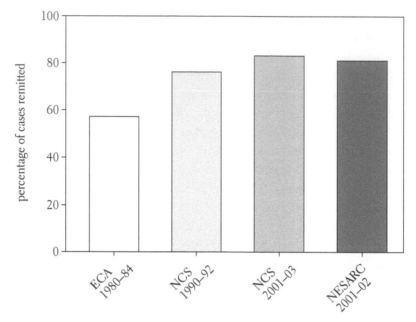

4.3 Drug disorder remission rates in the four largest nationwide scientific surveys. Besides the ECA and the first NCS, there are two additional data sets in this figure: the second NCS, 2001–2003 (Kessler et al., 2005a, 2005b), and NESARC, sponsored by the NIAAA (Stinson et al., 2005).

clinical texts, addiction research papers, and government bulletins for public education. That the four largest, most methodologically rigorous studies of psychiatric disorders and their correlates fail to support the claim is surprising. Surprising results require a higher standard of proof, ideally from studies that use different methods. The next two studies provide information on relapse but do not involve the same anonymous, one-interview approach of the large surveys. These subjects were interviewed repeatedly, and the researchers made use of either metabolic tests or "third-party" observers to validate the information obtained in the interviews.

Remission rates in studies with validated self-reports. Lee Robins, who is one of the primary organizers of the ECA project and a major contributor to the scientific transformation of psychiatry, conducted two studies that provide data on recovery in drug users that were selected independent of drug treatment. The first of the two projects was conducted in St. Louis (Robins & Murphy, 1967). The subjects were selected on the basis of having attended elementary schools in a neighborhood in which heroin was easy to obtain. Since drug use did not start until the boys were considerably older, their participation in the research project was independent of treatment and also independent of drug use itself. Nevertheless, by early adulthood about 15 percent of the boys had used heroin at least once. Of this group, about 75 percent became addicted, typically using at least several times a week. This was confirmed by official records. For instance, most of the subjects who said they were addicted to heroin were known to the local branch of a federal agency responsible for prosecuting addicts. However, when the men were in their early thirties, these same official sources reported that no more than 25 percent of those who had been addicted were still active cases. By self-report about 15 percent of those once addicted had used heroin in the last year (and this may have been a more up-to-date estimate). These results fit those of the large surveys, but the sample is extremely small, only twenty-two heroin addicts. The second study makes up for the size deficit.

As the Vietnam War was ending, Lee Robins was selected by President Nixon's Special Action Office of Drug Abuse Prevention to head a high-priority study of drug use among soldiers stationed in Vietnam. This was prompted by reports that large numbers of enlistees were using heroin. In light of the understandings of the day, the news was particularly disturbing. The Nixon administration feared a drug-fueled crime wave upon the soldiers' return from Vietnam. Then, as now, it was widely held that addiction was a chronic, relapsing disorder, that heroin was probably the most addictive of all drugs, and that to support their ever-increasing drug appetites, heroin addicts would turn to crime. In the early 1970s thousands of enlisted men were returning from Vietnam each month. Compounding the dire predictions, the country was experiencing the tail ends of the drug and crime "epidemics" of the 1960s. The returning servicemen, driven by cravings for heroin, familiar with violence and weapons, promised to bring both back to life.

Robins and her colleagues managed to recruit more than 400 opiate-using returning soldiers (which may make it the largest study of heroin users) who met the study's criteria for addiction (Robins, 1993; Robins et al., 1975; Robins et al., 1980). They used opiates on a regular basis, they experienced withdrawal symptoms, and they claimed that they were addicted. Most snorted or smoked heroin, a sign that the heroin was not as adulterated as in the United States. Some injected heroin, however, and the percentage of those who injected increased as a function of number of months in Vietnam, implying greater tolerance to opiates. In keeping with the signs of addiction, there were also signs of what is usually called "compulsive" use. When it was time to go home, many of the enlistees kept using heroin on a daily or near-daily basis, even though they knew they would be tested for opiates and that a positive result would delay their trip home. When queried about this, they said they couldn't stop because they were addicted. Thus, if heroin addiction is chronic, we would expect the enlistees to keep sniffing or injecting heroin when they returned home.

Back in the United States, no more than 12 percent of those who had been addicted while in Vietnam resumed use at a level that met the study's criteria for addiction. Urine samples corroborated the interview data. Those who said they were still current heroin users tested positive; those who said they didn't use heroin tested negative. Note also that for about 50 percent of the enlistees, drug use while in Vietnam was also confirmed by drug-positive urine samples.

The St. Louis and Vietnam studies are similar to the large surveys presented earlier in that the subjects were recruited independently of whether they were in treatment. But otherwise, their methods differed. In the two smaller studies, the relationship between the researchers and the interviewees was more intimate. There were urine tests and third-party verification of drug use. The subjects were in their late twenties or early thirties, so that errors of memory were less likely to affect the results. Nevertheless, the findings were the same as in the large, retrospective surveys. Most of those who were heavy illicit drug users and met the researchers' criteria for addiction stopped using or greatly cut down on heroin after a few years. This is also the picture of addiction that emerged from the biographies presented in Chapter 3.

Replication is the gold standard for scientific findings. By this criterion, addiction is not chronic. Indeed, it could be said that it is just the opposite: self-limiting. Note that nothing has been said about treatment. This is because most of those who quit were not in treatment. Together the two findings suggest that addiction is not a chronic disorder, but a limited and, after some years, perhaps, a self-correcting disorder.

Is Remission Forever?

Given that heavy drug use typically starts in the late teens or early twenties and that the median age in the large surveys was about 41 years old, the simplest conclusion is that most addicts stopped using drugs at high levels in their late twenties or early thirties. The biographical accounts of addiction and the research by Lee Robins also lead to this conclusion. However, there is an alternative account. It is not as simple but it has the advantage of preserving the claim that addiction is a chronic disorder. Imagine that addiction involves a cycling back and forth between periods of abstinence and periods of heavy drug use, and then add the qualification that the periods of abstinence persist much longer than the periods of heavy drug use. Given this temporal pattern, in a survey that interviewed subjects just once, the occasional yet enduring heavy drug users would look like they were ex-addicts—rather than occasional yet chronic addicts. This pattern explains the results and does not call for a revision of widely held understandings of addiction.

The idea that addiction consists of relatively short periods of heavy drug use followed by relatively longer periods of abstinence is easily tested. It predicts that one-time surveys will show that the overall rate of addiction remains approximately constant as a function of age. The next graph, Figure 4.4, tests this prediction. The data are from two of the major surveys (the ECA and first NCS) so that it is possible to check the reliability of the findings. On the horizontal axis is age. On the vertical axis is the percentage of currently active cases of addiction. If those who met the criteria for addiction when they were younger but did not do so at the time of survey have quit for good, then the data should show a downward trend. On the other hand, if "quitting" is actually part of a recurring cycle and terminates in relapse, the data points should remain more or less at the same level as a function of age.

For both cohorts, the age trend is sharply decreasing, suggesting that when those who met the criteria for lifetime drug dependence quit, they usually quit for good.[2] Also note that the decrease is steepest between the ages of 20 and 30, which is the prediction based on the biographical accounts given in the last chapter. That both cohorts show the same pattern suggests that the results are not an historical quirk but reflect a general feature of addiction. The biographical accounts suggested that most addicts quit drugs by their early thirties, and the epidemiological data strongly support this suggestion. To be sure, addicts may relapse the first few times they try to quit, but, according to the surveys, by about age 30 most have quit for good. Thus, for addiction, quitting drugs is more accurately described as "resolution," not "remission," when the ex-drug user is more than 30 years old.

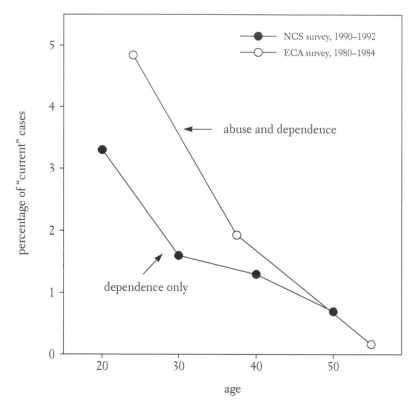

4.4 Persistence of addiction as a function of age. Data are from the ECA and the first NCS.

Making Sense of the Survey Data and Received Knowledge

The simplest explanation of the discrepancy between the research findings and received knowledge regarding the nature of addiction is that experts are basing their understanding of addiction on addicts who show up in the treatment clinics, whereas the research reviewed in this chapter is based on studies that selected subjects independent of treatment history, with the goal of obtaining a representative sample. Both approaches would lead to similar results if most addicts ended up in treatment. But most addicts do not seek treatment. Given that the clinic studies support the claim that addiction is a chronic disorder, this means that addicts who end up in treatment keep using drugs, treatment notwithstanding, and those not in treatment quit using drugs. This interpretation fits all the data presented so far, and it also suggests an interesting hypothesis.

Although addiction studies that select subjects independent of treatment show high recovery rates, some of those who meet the criteria for substance dependence will have been in treatment. In contrast to the overall trends shown in Figures 4.1 to 4.4, the addicts who were in treatment will still meet the criteria for dependence—or at least to a greater extent than addicts who were never in treatment. Relapse rates in Vietnam veterans who were addicted to opiates and sought treatment provide a perfect test of this hypothesis.

About 14 percent of the veterans who met the criteria for opiate addiction sought treatment when they returned to the United States. Robins interviewed these men and was able to determine if and when they re lapsed following treatment for addiction. Figure 4.5 shows the results. On the horizontal axis is the number of weeks since the end of treatment. As predicted, the Vietnam veterans in treatment had higher relapse rates

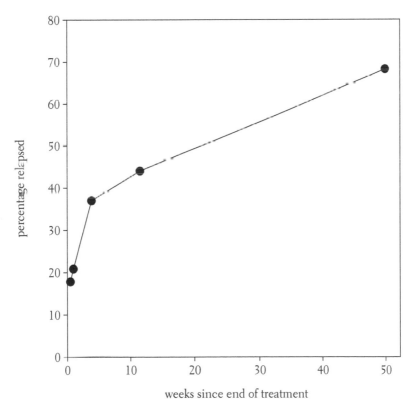

weeks since end of treatment

4.5 Relapse rate for the Vietnam veteran opiate users who sought treatment. Addiction is much more likely to be a relapsing disorder for addicts who seek treatment. Data are from Robins, 1993.

than those who were not in treatment. Indeed, the relapse rate for the clinic Vietnam veterans exceeded that of their nonclinic peers by more than a factor of five.[3]

Why Are Remission Rates So Different in the Clinic and General Population Studies?

The finding that addicts in treatment were more likely to relapse than those not in treatment often triggers the following exchange: "Those in treatment were more addicted." "What do you mean by more addicted?" "They used drugs longer." What is missing here is an account of why those in treatment used drugs longer. This has not been studied much, most likely because it has been widely believed that addicts in treatment did better than those not in treatment. There are some data, however, and they provide information on two important hypotheses. First, it is reasonable to suppose that differences in pharmacological history distinguish the two groups. Second, it is just as plausible that individual differences distinguish the two groups. These are not mutually exclusive explanations and both promise to increase our understanding of the determinants of drug use in addicts.

The difference in relapse rates could be due to pharmacological factors. For instance, clinic addicts might use more addictive drugs. In support of this hypothesis, many clinics specialize in heroin addiction (e.g., methadone clinics), but few if any clinics specialize in marijuana addiction. However, implicit in the pharmacological account is the assumption that relapse varies markedly as a function of type of drug. This may not be true. For example, if mounting costs is one of the factors that brings drug use to a halt, then heroin addicts would be more likely to abstain than marijuana addicts (all else being equal). Thus, we should first test whether there are drug-based differences in the persistence of drug use. Figure 4.6 summarizes the relevant data for the two largest community surveys (Anthony & Helzer, 1991; Stinson et al., 2005).

The graph shows that the remission rates for the three drug classes did not differ markedly. The implication is that the higher remission rates for clinic addicts is not a function of using drugs that are more addictive. The results, though, may seem discrepant with findings discussed in Chapter 2. Recall that the likelihood that drug use led to dependence was substantially higher for heroin than for cocaine, and the addiction rate for cocaine was higher than the addiction rate for marijuana (Figure

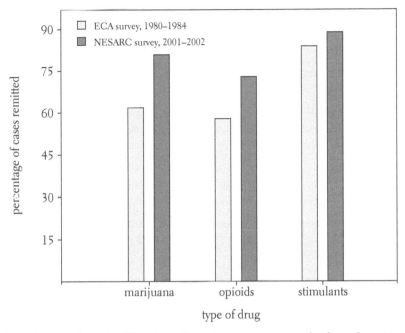

4.6 Remission rates for major illicit drugs. Remission rates were somewhat lower for opiates and higher for stimulants, but the differences were not large. Data are from the ECA (Anthony & Helzer, 1991) and NESARC (Stinson et al., 2005).

2.2). The simplest interpretation is that the factors associated with the etiology of addiction differ from the factors that influence the persistence of addiction. Pharmacology appears to play a larger role in the transition from use to abuse than it does in quitting, whereas individual differences, such as those correlated with treatment, appear to play a larger role in quitting than in onset. In any case, given that remission rate did not vary much with type of drug, the data imply that type of drug cannot explain why addicts in clinics are more likely to relapse than addicts not in clinics. When it comes to quitting, type of drug does not explain much.

Do quantitative differences in drug use explain higher clinic relapse rates? Perhaps the clinic populations tend to use illicit drugs longer because they started using drugs at a younger age or used them more frequently once they became heavy users. That is, greater pharmacological exposure could explain why clinic addicts are much more likely to persist in drug use than nonclinic addicts. Two studies, both conducted by Yale

Medical School researchers, provide data relevant to this hypothesis. One study focused on opiate users (Rounsaville & Kleber, 1985); the other focused on cocaine users (Carroll & Rounsaville, 1992). In both projects, the clinic and community subjects were about the same age.

In the heroin study, drug exposure was measured in terms of age of onset, duration, and frequency. By these measures the community and treatment populations did not differ. For both groups the average age of onset was 18 years old. For both groups, heavy use was ongoing for about six years, and for both groups, the frequency of heroin use averaged out to between 22 and 23 days per month. But there were significant differences when it came to other drugs. The community (nonclinic) addicts scored about twice as high on the Michigan Alcoholism Screening Test, and they used marijuana, hallucinogens, and inhalants more often. Thus, the two groups used opiates to about the same extent, but those in treatment had less exposure to other drugs.

The cocaine study produced similar results. Treatment and nontreatment cocaine addicts did not differ in terms of level of cocaine use. Both groups started using cocaine at about age eighteen, both had been using regularly for about three to four years, and both groups used at about the same rate—fifteen days a month. However, as in the opiate study, those not in treatment were more likely to also abuse other drugs.

Comorbidity Predicts Relapse

The available evidence fails to support a pharmacological explanation of why addicts in treatment are less likely to quit using drugs. However, it should be pointed out that there are very few published papers that compare clinic and nonclinic drug users. Perhaps if this topic were studied more intensively, differences in pharmacological history or pharmacological response would emerge.

In contrast, it has proved easy to find individual differences that are correlated with differences in treatment history. The most important is that addicts in treatment are much more likely to suffer from additional psychiatric disorders than those not in treatment. In the ECA survey the ratio was more than two to one (Regier et al., 1990). About 64 percent of those in the clinics suffered from at least one additional psychiatric disorder, whereas for those who said they had not sought clinic help for drug use, the comorbidity rate was about 30 percent, a number that is closer to

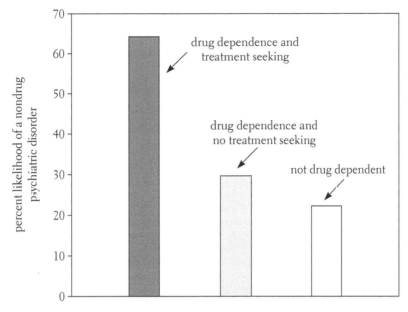

4.7 The relationships between addiction, treatment, and additional psychiatric disorders. Individuals who met the criteria for a drug disorder were more than twice as likely to seek treatment if they also met the criteria for an additional psychiatric disorder. Data are from the ECA survey; Regier et al., 1990.

the psychiatric prevalence rate for nonaddicts (see Figure 4.7). The more recent and larger NIAAA survey reports similar results (Stinson et al., 2005), as do smaller studies. For instance, in two reports from drug clinics associated with Yale Medical School, the rate of comorbidity for cocaine and heroin addicts was 74 and 87 percent, respectively (Rounsaville et al., 1991; Rounsaville et al., 1982).

Although the comorbidity rates for clinic addicts are quite high, they may actually underestimate the true differences between clinic and non-clinic populations. This is because comorbidity analyses have been re-stricted to psychiatric disorders, whereas heavy drug users often suffer from a variety of nonpsychiatric medical ailments as well. For instance, those who inject cocaine and heroin almost always carry the hepatitis C virus and often carry the AIDS virus as well. In addition many illicit-drug addicts who visit clinics are heavy drinkers with various drinking-related health problems. These ailments do not count in the comorbidity studies. Moreover, the studies use a simple dichotomous scale of "present" or "not present," whereas actual disorders vary continuously. Thus, there are good reasons for thinking that the health of clinic-treated addicts is actually substantially worse than the available literature suggests.

Why does comorbidity predict relapse? Edward Khantzian, a Boston psychiatrist and psychoanalyst, argued that addiction was actually a self-medication process (e.g., 1997). According to this idea, addicts use drugs to solve their predrug psychological problems. For instance, someone who is overwrought with feelings of anger and resentment will take drugs that temper his hostility, such as heroin. The theory is certainly plausible and is supported by the comorbidity data. A qualification, though, is in order. Figure 4.7 showed that the frequency of an additional psychiatric disorder for nonclinic addicts was not much greater than the frequency of one or more psychiatric disorders in the general, nonaddict population. That is, comorbidity was much more common in clinic than in nonclinic addicts. This finding takes on added significance when it is joined with the observation that addicts who have been in treatment are much more likely to remain addicts than those not in treatment. The immediate implication is that comorbidity is more strongly linked to the persistence of drug use than it is to its onset, and in turn this relationship suggests that the persistence of addiction into middle age is due largely to the presence of additional psychiatric disorders. The biographies help explain why additional psychiatric disorders sabotage the efforts of those who are trying to quit drugs.

According to the biographies, financial and family concerns were among the main reasons addicts quit using drugs. Economics and family responsibilities are also the concerns of adulthood. This suggests that the pressures that typically accompany "maturity" bring drug use to a halt in many addicts. Assuming this to be the case, then one of the reasons that comorbidity promotes drug use in addicts is that it gets in the way of adult roles. It seems reasonable to suppose that those who are very depressed or very anxious are less likely to be engaged in activities that are incompatible with heavy drug use. Put another way, psychiatric impairment renders the drug experience relatively more valuable by undermining the ability to engage in and enjoy competing activities. The more general message is that whether addicts keep using drugs or quit depends to a great extent on their alternatives. The remainder of this chapter and the subsequent chapters on choice provide findings and a theory that support this conclusion.

Fitting the Pieces Together: The Natural History of Addiction in Clinic and Nonclinic Addicts

The data on remission, clinic and nonclinic heavy drug users, and co-morbidity fit together like the pieces of a jigsaw puzzle. Most of those who meet the criteria for substance dependence start using illicit drugs in their late teens or early twenties, but then stop or greatly reduce their drug intake by their late twenties. Those who do not quit fill the rosters of the drug-treatment clinic. Although their histories differ from those of most addicts, their biographies are the ones that have informed clinical texts and expert opinion on the nature of addiction. According to the few studies that directly compared clinic and nonclinic drug users, those in treatment were much more likely to suffer from additional psychiatric and other medical disorders. Psychiatric and nonpsychiatric medical problems create barriers. They make it less likely for drug users to become involved in viable alternatives to drug use. Hence, the clinic drug addicts remain heavy drug users for much longer than the nonclinic heavy drug users. Surprisingly, it was not possible to document differences in pharmacological history for clinic and nonclinic addicts (holding age constant). The simplest summary of these observations is that addiction persists as a function of the addict's ability to take advantage of nondrug competing activities. Those with greater access to meaningful alternatives are more likely to quit using. This generalization is, of course, a way of saying that drug use in addicts is voluntary, or, put the other way around, addicts are not compulsive drug users; addiction is not a disease. However, as will be discussed in the next chapter, there may be good reasons for calling addiction a disease even if drug use in addicts persists as a function of budgetary concerns, meaningful alternatives, personal values, and the other variables that influence choice.

Clinics Can Help

This chapter began with textbook and journal article summaries of the results from treatment follow-up studies. The message was that success rates were low. However, the texts and articles failed to add that most addicts are not in treatment. The texts and articles also failed to point out that certain treatments do have a very good track record. These results deserve attention. They show clinicians what does work, and they provide insight into the nature of addiction. Figure 4.8 provides a sampling of the clinic success stories.

The graph shows that recovery, not relapse, hovered around the 80 to 90 percent mark. This is virtually the opposite of the findings emphasized by the clinical texts and general articles on addiction that have appeared in journals like *Science* and the *Lancet*. The different results correspond to differences in the treatment plans. For the patients shown in this graph—physicians and airplane pilots—relapse threatened their careers. These doctors and pilots could have lost their jobs if they resumed drug use. Moreover, to insure adherence, most of the treatment programs randomly tested their patients. Voucher programs that offer positive rewards also report successful outcomes, but not as high as these (e.g., Higgins et al., 1994, 2000). Together, the two approaches show that when there are relatively immediate and salient consequences for reducing drug use, ad-

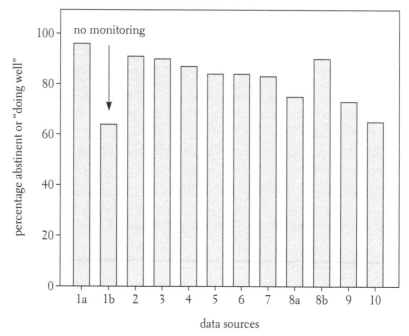

4.8 Abstinence rates for contingency-based drug treatment programs. The drug users were physicians and airplane pilots. In all but one program (1b), there were drug tests. Positive results could result in job loss. The numbers in the graph identify the publication that provided the data. Most of the studies are reviewed in Coombs, 1997. (1a and 1b) Shore, 1987; (2) Ganley et al., 2005; (3) Bohigian, 2005; (4) Flynn et al., 1993; (5) Paris & Canavan, 1999; (6) Gallegos & Norton, 1984; (7) Morse et al., 1984; (8) Domino et al., 2005; (9) Crowley, 1986; (10) Johnson & Connelly, 1981.

dicts comply. Interestingly, the consequences can be negative, as when one's career is under threat, or positive, as when the vouchers can be used to purchase household goods and access to recreational activities. Another common feature of the contingency, choice-based treatment results is that they are not as well known as the clinic failures.

Most of the studies that were discussed in this chapter were sponsored by NIH research grants and were conducted by well-recognized experts. The results appeared in widely read professional journals. Nevertheless, the findings did not support the words that introduce textbook and journal articles on addiction. They did not show that addiction was a "chronic, relapsing disease." In fact, addiction was the DSM disorder that had the highest resolution rate. To be sure, relapse is common in many clinic follow-up studies, but as just shown, there are notable exceptions. Moreover, it is common knowledge that clinic populations may provide a distorted picture of the natural history of a disorder. This bias even has a name: Berkson's bias. One possible explanation for the discrepancy between the research and widely accepted views on the nature of addiction is that ideas about addiction reflect habits of mind regarding drug effects and choice rather than the research. For instance, on the basis of widely shared ideas and a few facts, it is possible to create a story that addiction must be chronic. The line of reasoning goes like this: Self-destructive behavior implies sickness. Addiction is self-destructive, therefore it is an illness. If it is an illness, then the only way to get better is to seek help at a clinic. But addicts who get help at clinics do not get better; they keep using drugs. Therefore, all addicts, those in the clinic and those out, must keep using drugs, which is to say, addiction is a "chronic, relapsing disease."

This is a perfectly sensible line of reasoning, and it would yield a valid picture of the world if self-destructive behavior implies illness, and if those addicts who participated in the treatment studies were representative of addicts in general. However, those in the clinic are not representative, and in Chapters 6 and 7, it is shown that voluntary actions can be consistently self-destructive.

A critical step in this misguided argument is the notion that self-destructive behavior implies illness. If this is true then addicts should be eligible for benefits, such as disability insurance. This is an interesting as well as an important issue. For instance, given the number of addicts, disability payments would be very expensive. Of course, the matter should be decided on a balanced and fair sampling of the research results, not what is believed to be true or a selective sampling of studies that we know are not representative of the general population of addicts. The following chapter takes up these issues. One of the findings is that the disease interpretation follows as a natural consequence of widely held ideas regarding individual responsibility and free will.

5

VOLUNTARY BEHAVIOR, DISEASE, AND ADDICTION

In 1818 Samuel Judd, a New York whale-oil merchant, was summoned to court for refusing to pay the city fish-oil tax (Burnett, 2007). Judd refused on the grounds that a whale is not a fish. Experts testified on the anatomy of whale sexual organs, their mating behavior, parenting, how they breathe, and skeletal structure. According to these behavioral, physiological, and anatomical features, whales were more like dogs and even humans than tuna and sardines. But the jury understood that fish were animals that lived in the sea and mammals were animals that lived on land. Since whales lived in the sea, a whale was a fish. Indeed, unless Mr. Judd could show that whales lived on land, he had to pay the fish-oil tax. The jury was aware that mother whales nursed baby whales, but this did not count as much as the long-held classification schemes that fish were water animals, mammals were land animals, and birds flew in the air.

The story is instructive. It shows that arguments about how to classify a phenomenon can reflect different understandings of the basic terms as much as the particular features of the phenomenon in question. No one mentioned that a fish has a two-chambered heart, whereas a whale has a four-chambered heart with two ventricles, just like cows and other mammals. Rather the differences in opinion concerned the criteria for distinguishing mammals and fish. One school of thought based the distinction on habitat, the other based the distinction on physiological characteristics. This chapter makes a similar point regarding the classification of addiction. It shows that scientific explanations for why addiction should be considered a disease depend on assumptions regarding the relevant categories, which in this case are involuntary and voluntary behaviors. For example, one of the mainstays of the claim that addiction is a disease is evidence that it has a genetic basis. The idea is that if genes influence an activity, then it can't be voluntary. There are, however, everyday experiences which suggest that even clearly voluntary activities have a genetic basis. As children get older, they often find themselves adopting attitudes that are more and more like those of their parents, even when they have moved far away and don't particularly appreciate the similarities. Attitudes are learned, but aspects of this common experience suggest that genes are also at play. Thus, we need to check if genetic differences play an important role in voluntary activities. If so, then a genetic basis for addiction does not automatically mean that addicts are "compulsive, involuntary" drug users. Put more generally, if a key feature of a disease state is that the symptoms are involuntary, then we need to know how to distinguish between voluntary and involuntary behavior.

What Sort of Disease Is Addiction?

In the preface to *Alcoholics Anonymous* (1939), Dr. W. D. Silkworth suggests that alcoholics have an "allergy." The allergen is alcohol, and the allergic reaction is loss of control over drinking. One drink leads to another drink, which leads to another, just as ragweed pollen initiates a fit of sneezing. In recent years the allergy model of addiction has expanded to include many other involuntary medical states. In clinical texts and scientific journals, researchers say that addiction should be grouped with such diseases as Alzheimer's, hypertension, Type 2 diabetes, schizophrenia, asthma, arthritis, and even cancer and heart disease (e.g., Leshner, 1997; McLellan et al., 2000; O'Brien & McLellan, 1996; USDHHS, 2007). If these comparisons are apt, then it is cruel and unjust to subject those who meet the criteria for dependence to criminal charges or even criticism. This would be like scolding someone with Alzheimer's for getting lost or reprimanding a Tourette's syndrome patient for gesticulating wildly. In this vein, Dr. Enoch Gordis (1995), a champion of science-based alcoholism treatment and previous head of NIAAA, writes: "the disease concept . . . has helped remove the stigma from a chronic disorder [alcoholism] that is no more inherently immoral than diabetes or heart disease." Taking this argument to its logical conclusion, a group of leading addiction researchers argued (in the pages of the *Journal of the American Medical Association*) that insurance plans should provide the same coverage for heroin addiction, crack addiction, and alcoholism as they do for traditional chronic diseases such as cancer, arthritis, and high blood pressure (McLellan et al., 2000). Although this may seem a radical (and expensive) proposal, if addiction is a disease, it is not unreasonable.

Why Addiction Is a Disease

Although it will be shown that intuitions regarding the nature of voluntary behavior prove to be the foundation for the disease interpretation of addiction, there are also important empirical arguments to consider. These have appeared in scholarly and scientific venues, such as psychiatric handbooks, journal articles, and clinic mission statements. They typically focus on three lines of evidence and reasoning: (1) addiction has a biological basis; (2) addictive drugs have the capacity to transform a voluntary user into an involuntary one; and (3) the disease interpretation leads to better treatment for addicts. These views will be discussed in turn.

IS THERE A GENETIC PREDISPOSITION FOR ADDICTION?

At the NIDA-sponsored College on Problems of Drug Dependence meetings in 2003, which is the major conference for addiction researchers, there was a symposium on the disease interpretation of addiction. At the end of the talks, someone in the audience stated that addiction was a disease "because it has a genetic basis, and we do not choose our genes." This is a succinct summary of an idea that is broadly endorsed by scientists and nonscientists alike. In discussions of addiction, the claim that addicts choose to get high is often countered with the point, "But there is a genetic predisposition for alcoholism." This response encompasses two important ideas. The first is that addiction has a genetic basis; the second is that if an activity is influenced by genes, it is not correct to say that it is voluntary. Let's first check if it is really true that genes can influence whether someone becomes an addict.

Genetics and addiction. Most of the research on the role of genetics in drug use has focused on alcoholics. This is because it is easier to conduct multi-generational research on legal drugs than on illegal ones. The basic finding is that alcoholism runs in families, and this is true even when the family members did not live together. Dr. Robert Cloninger (1987) led a project that nicely illustrates the genetic approach to the study of alcoholism. The research was carried out in Sweden, a country in which adoption was not uncommon, and in which the biological and nonbiological parents' drinking histories were on record.

The subjects were men who had been given up for adoption at an average age of 4 months. This population was of special interest to researchers, because the Swedish social service agencies had detailed records of not only the boys, but their biological parents and their adoptive parents. In particular much was known about the drinking histories of all parties. According to the agency records, there were about 1,700 adoptees that had developed drinking problems, with about half meeting the criteria for "severe" alcohol abuse and half meeting the criteria for "less severe" alcohol abuse.

The major finding was that the biological father's drinking pattern was a better predictor of alcohol abuse in the adopted son than the father by adoption's drinking pattern. For instance, the rates of alcoholism for boys whose biological fathers were severe alcoholics were nearly identical regardless of whether their adoptive father was an alcoholic or teetotaler. For those who grew up in a home with an alcoholic (adoptive) father, the rate of alcoholism was 18 percent; for those who grew up in a home free of parental alcoholism, the rate was 17 percent. That is, given that the biological father was a severe alcoholic, parental drinking patterns did not matter.

Studies of the genetics of illicit drug use yield similar findings. The researchers, though, typically compared twins rather than following adoptees. In a representative example of the twin approach, Dr. Kenneth Kendler and his colleagues at the Medical College of Virginia and Virginia Commonwealth University (2000) tabulated the correlations in illegal drug use and illegal drug addiction for fraternal and identical twins. Their hypothesis was that if there was a genetic basis for addiction, then the correlations among identical twins would be significantly greater than those for fraternal twins. The results for addiction supported the genetic hypothesis but not the results for use, which includes experimentation that did not proceed to addiction. For identical and fraternal twins, the correlations were nearly identical for simple use. If one twin had experimented with an illicit drug, then there was about a 75 percent chance that the other had as well. That is, number of shared genes did not influence the correlations for experimenting with illegal drugs. In contrast, the correlations for drug addiction varied as a function of the percentage of shared genes. If one member of a fraternal twin pair had been dependent, then there was about a 25 percent chance that his co-twin was also dependent; whereas if one member of an identical twin pair was dependent, then there was a 40 percent chance that his identical brother was also dependent. When the number of shared genes was doubled, there was more than a 50 percent increase in between-twin similarity for addiction. Dr. Ming Tsuang and his colleagues at Harvard Medical School have conducted similar studies with twins who were in the military during the Vietnam War (1998). Their results are similar to those of the Virginia study.

There can be little doubt that genes can play an important role in the etiology of addiction. But does this mean in these cases, drug use has become involuntary? We can answer this question by asking whether genes also play a role in activities that are voluntary. If they do, then genetic influences do not preclude choice. But before I present some relevant data on this topic, notice that the correlation for addiction among identical twins was far less than 100 percent and that fewer than 20 percent of the biological sons of serious alcoholics became alcoholics themselves, even when their adoptive fathers were alcoholics. These facts say that the pathway from DNA to addiction is indirect, with genes programming proteins that affect the probability of addiction rather than insuring that it does or does not occur. The same point is made by a more general consideration.

We inherit genes; we do not inherit behaviors. As a function of a variety of factors that come under the term "gene expression" and which include behavioral and environmental influences, genes make proteins. Differences in the proteins lead to differences in behavior, but since the genes make proteins, not behaviors, the genetic influences are indirect. In the case of alcohol, the following pathways are well documented: metabolism (e.g., Luczak et al., 2001), antisocial behavior (Haber et al., 2005), and tolerance (Schuckit, 1994). Presumably, there are other pathways as well. But none include DNA-programmed behavioral modules for shooting up or going to the store to buy a six-pack. Rather, genes are one of the various factors that exercise some influence over drug-seeking and drug self-administration. Indeed what they do, albeit indirectly, is affect the relative value of alcohol. If a genetic difference makes alcohol toxic, then you are less likely to prefer alcohol.

Do genes also influence voluntary activities? The famous Charles Addams cartoon of the separated-at-birth Mallifert twins showing up at the same time in the same patent attorney's office hoping to get a patent for the identical gizmos sitting on their respective laps suggests that everyday life offers plenty of evidence that voluntary activities are influenced by genes. In recent years, researchers have caught up with intuition. They have examined the role of heredity in social attitudes, such as support for the death penalty and whether women should have non-domestic professions (Bouchard et al., 2003; Tesser & Crelia, 1994). One of the most interesting studies evaluated the role of genes in religious beliefs. Religious beliefs are learned and voluntary. In early adulthood, many people question their faith, sometimes discarding the beliefs they grew up with and replacing them with new ones. Conversely, those who keep their faith often reaffirm it after encountering situations that question the ideas they learned as children. Thus, religious beliefs provide a powerful test of the role of genes in voluntary behavior. If heredity influences beliefs about a deity, then it is hard to imagine voluntary actions that are not to some degree influenced by heredity.

The next graph reports the results of a study on religious beliefs in twins (Waller et al., 1990). The twins grew up in different families and were separated before the age of one year. Religious beliefs and behavior were assessed by questionnaires that identified the informants' thoughts about the nature of God, the role of prayer in their lives, and the literal accuracy of Bible stories. The results are summarized in Figure 5.1. The black bars show the level of agreement between identical twins; the grey bars show the level of agreement between fraternal twins. Identical twins often agreed with each other; fraternal twins agreed at about a chance level. But neither the identical nor the fraternal twins grew up together. They grew up in different families. These results do not stand alone. There are now many studies on the heritability of attitudes and beliefs, and they typically show that beliefs reflect genetic as well as familial and cultural influences (e.g., Olson et al., 2001; Rutherford et al., 1993). Religious beliefs are voluntary; genes affect religious beliefs; genes affect voluntary behavior.

DO DRUG-INDUCED BRAIN CHANGES ESTABLISH ADDICTION AS A DISEASE?

The last few decades have witnessed remarkable advances in techniques that provide information on the structure and functioning of the brain. It is now possible to visualize the brain under a wide range of conditions and undertakings, including cognitive tasks, decision-making tasks, participation in situations that elicit emotions such as sympathy, and drug self-administration. The drug studies have shed new light on how drugs work (e.g., Lukas & Renshaw, 1998). They have also been adopted by

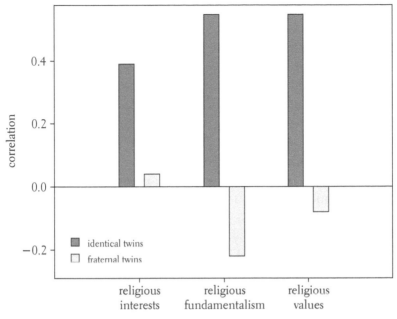

5.1 The correlation between religious values and heredity in fraternal and identical twins who were raised apart. Data are from Waller et al., 1990

those interested in classifying addiction as a disease, and in recent years have become the primary pillar for the claim that addiction is a disease. Alan Leshner, director of NIDA from 1994 until 2001, put the case most succinctly in a review paper published in *Science* (1997). "That addiction is tied to changes in brain structure and function is what makes it, fundamentally, a disease." Glen Hanson, Leshner's immediate successor at NIDA, makes the same point in slightly different words (Hanson et al., 2002): "Almost three decades of research [shows that] drug addiction comes about as a result of the long-lasting effects of drugs on brain function. Therefore we say it is a brain disease." Supporting that argument, *NIDA InfoFacts*, a U.S. government public health bulletin, reports (June, 2008): "Drug addiction is a *brain disease* because the abuse of drugs leads to changes in the structure and function of the brain" (NIDA 2008, p. 1, emphasis theirs).

That drugs change the brain is a logical necessity as well as experimental fact. Drugs change behavior, mood, and thought; the brain is the organ of behavior, mood, and thought; thus drugs change the brain. Over the last ten years or so, hundreds of experimental reports support this logic (e.g., Lukas & Renshaw, 1998; Nestler et al., 1993; Robinson et al., 2001; Volkow et al., 1990). Yet, as was the case for the genetic argument, it only makes sense to say that drug-induced changes in brain function are proof that a disorder is a disease if certain other conditions are met. For genetics, the critical other condition was that genes did not influence voluntary behaviors. By the same logic, drug-induced brain changes are sufficient evidence that addiction is a disease if neural plasticity is not associated with voluntary acts. But it is obvious that the factors that influence voluntary behavior do so by changing the brain. Neural plasticity is what makes voluntary behavior possible. In support of this point are hundreds of studies documenting that changes in voluntary activities are associated with changes in the brain (see, for example, recent introductory psychology texts, e.g., Bernstein et al., 2005; Gazzaniga & Heatherton, 2006; Schacter et al., 2009). Many of these studies are directly relevant to addiction because they help explain why addiction can have such high recovery rates. A study on brain plasticity and obsessive-compulsive disorder (OCD) helps make the connections between brain plasticity, voluntary behavior, and recovery clear.

Brain plasticity as an opportunity for recovery. Individuals with OCD are plagued by disturbing thoughts. They find temporary relief by engaging in ritualized behaviors that address their obsessions. For example, the idea that one's hands are swarming with infectious bacteria can be put to rest by washing. But then the thought returns, and with it, the motivation to wash one's hands returns. Therapists have developed behavioral and cognitive techniques that help OCD patients ignore their disturbing thoughts. Follow-up studies show that these techniques are quite effective (e.g., Seligman et al., 2001). This implies that the behavioral and cognitive techniques must have changed the brain. An interesting study by Jeffrey Schwartz, a psychiatrist who specializes in OCD treatment, confirmed this inference.

Schwartz and his colleagues taught OCD patients to ignore their obsessive thoughts (Schwartz, 1998). This led to a marked reduction in compulsive rituals and even a reduction in the intrusive thoughts. The researchers also measured neural activity in areas of the brain that are associated with OCD symptoms. For those patients who learned to ignore their obsessions, activity levels in the critical brain areas were now similar to those of OCD-free control subjects. Pharmacological agents that help ameliorate compulsive behavior produced similar changes in brain activity (Baxter et al., 1992). Summarizing these findings, Schwartz writes: "change your behavior, change your brain." This comment captures the dynamic quality of brain and behavior interactions, but it leaves out the fact that the patients had an incentive for changing their behavior. Thus, the more complete summary of the successful OCD treatment results is: "change the incentives, change your behavior, change your brain."

The OCD research is relevant to the stories of recovery in Chapter 3. Recall, for example, that Patty and Jessie learned to ignore their cravings for cocaine. Changes in their lives created new incentives to quit using drugs. Thus, when they experienced cocaine cravings, the urge to use drugs was in competition with the motives to pay bills, be a better parent, do better at work, and so on. As a result drug use decreased, and eventually the cravings themselves were extinguished. Although their stories say nothing explicit about their brains, on the basis of research such as the OCD study that was just described, it must be the case that Patty and Jessie's transition from heavy cocaine use was in part paved by the neural changes that accompanied their ability to ignore the cocaine cravings. If OCD patients can learn to ignore obsessional thought, then it seems reasonable that similar processes are taking place when addicts learn to ignore drug cravings. Thus, drug-induced brain change is not sufficient evidence that addiction is an involuntary disease state. Drugs change the brain, but this does not make addiction a disease.

ON THE CLAIM THAT BIOLOGICAL INFLUENCE IMPLIES THAT ADDICTION IS A DISEASE

Genes influence the etiology of addiction and addictive drugs alter the brain. However, we also saw that genes influence the etiology of voluntary behaviors and that brain plasticity is inherent to changes in voluntary behavior. The issue then is not whether genes or neuroadaptations influence drug use. Rather the key question is whether genes or neuroadaptations turn voluntary drug use into involuntary drug use. Or put another way, the debate about the nature of addiction has been framed as a biological issue, yet the biological data have not helped solve it. The reason is that the criteria for deciding whether an activity is voluntary are behavioral. We do not look at people's genes to determine if they are engaged in a voluntary or involuntary act, we look at their behavior. Similarly, we do not look at their brains to decide if their actions are voluntary or not. This is not to deny that there are biological underpinnings to the distinction between voluntary and involuntary acts. Rather, the point is that the distinction rests on criteria that precede what we have learned about the brain. Possibly a better set of criteria will emerge, but future developments cannot possibly be relevant to the current discussion of whether addiction is a disease. There is, however, some disagreement regarding the behavioral signs of voluntary and involuntary acts. Everyday language and thought offers one rule, which I will call the traditional rule, and research on behavior also offers a rule. Let's consider first the traditional understanding of voluntary action.

A Historical Sketch of the Understanding
of Voluntary Behavior and Addiction

Seventeenth-century understandings of addiction. Historical studies show that the idea that heavy drug use is a disease state preceded both biological science and any clear understanding of the relationship between the nervous system and behavior. We know this thanks to the detective work of Jessica Warner, a historian with an interest in addiction. In a paper titled "'Resolv'd to drink no more': Addiction as a preindustrial construct" (1994), she documents a series of texts that are likely the earliest known writings on addiction. The authors are members of the clergy, and the intended audience includes those who are or could become alcoholics.

In 1619, Robert Harris described habitual drunkenness as a "dropsilike disease." In 1622, Samuel Ward writes of the "drunkard's disease," and in 1628, William Prynne notes that drunkenness is a "dangerous dropsie and disease." ("Dropsie" referred to abnormal swelling in the soft tissues, which in many cases was probably a symptom of heart disease.) Moreover, "habitual drunkenness" had no cure and was spreading. John Bury (1677) writes that drunkenness is a disease "so epidemical" that "all the Physicians in *England* know not how to stop it."

The reasoning behind the clergy's belief that they were dealing with a disease is that their "sick" parishioners kept drinking despite drinking-related problems. John Downame, who died in 1652, put it this way: "The last spirtuall euill which the drunkard brigeth vpon himslefe, is finall impentencie; for they who addict themselues to this vice, doe finde it so sweete and plesaing to the flesh, that they are loth to part with it, and by long custome they turne delight into necessitie . . . and howsoeuer the manifold mischiefes into which they plunge themselues, serue as so manie forcible arguments to disswade them from this vice, yet against all rules of reason, they hold fast their conclusion, that come what come may, they will not leaue their drunkennes" (Downame, 1609, p. 101, cited in Warner, 1994, p. 687). Although the spellings are unfamiliar, the ideas are not. Drunkards kept drinking despite "the rules of reason" and despite the "manifold mischiefes into which they plunge themselues." This is the seventeenth-century version of the APA account of addiction: the persistence of drug use despite drug-related problems.

The seventeenth-century account of alcoholism is not based on biology but on widely shared understandings of voluntary behavior. The fundamental assumption is that individuals make choices that are in their best interests. Since addiction is self-destructive, the logical implication is that addicts cannot be voluntarily choosing to use drugs. Since the symptoms of diseases are involuntary, then addiction must be a disease. In other words, medical evidence did not turn alcoholism into a disease, but rather the assumption that voluntary behavior is not self-destructive turned alcoholism into a disease. Next, we will see that present-day addiction researchers make precisely the same argument, although with a somewhat different vocabulary (and spellings).

Current versions of the idea that addicts are involuntary drug users. In an article published in the journal *Science*, Alan Leshner (1997) equates addiction with compulsivity. Why one implies the other, however, is not explained. "A metaphorical switch in the brain seems to be thrown as a result of prolonged drug use. Initially, drug use is a voluntary behavior, but when that switch is thrown, the individual moves into the state of addiction characterized by compulsive drug seeking and use" (p. 46). The account is straightforward, except that the key term, "compulsive," is not defined. In the British medical journal *The Lancet*, O'Brien and McLellan (1996) draw similar connections: "At some point after continued repetition of voluntary drug taking, the drug 'user' loses the voluntary ability to control its use. At this point the drug 'misuser' becomes 'drug addicted' and there is a compulsive, often overwhelming *involuntary* aspect to continued drug use" (p. 237). O'Brien and McLellan make much the same point as Leshner. In this passage, "addicted" means compulsive and involuntary. Neither they nor Leshner define what they mean by "compulsive" and "involuntary," nor do they say why addiction implies compulsivity. It is as if to say "addicted" is to say "involuntary." Miller and Chappel, two psychiatrists who have written one of the most comprehensive and useful accounts of the disease interpretation of drug dependence, "History of the disease concept" (1991), put voluntariness at the heart of addiction: "Rarely overtly stated but clearly central to the concept of a disease is a victim state. As a victim, the afflicted has no control over the progression of the disease if left untreated. In the disease concept of alcoholism (and drug addiction), the cardinal feature is *loss of control* over the use of alcohol . . . The loss of control, which can actually be inherited, is the sine qua non for alcoholism (and drug addiction) as qualifying for the disease state. The loss of control signifies a victim that reflects an alteration of brain function" (p. 197).

These passages are linked by the common idea that, by definition, addiction is involuntary drug use and also by the common practice of not defining the key terms. Although the quotations are taken from science journals, none of the authors, nor, presumably, the editors or reviewers, considered it necessary to define what they meant by "loss of control," "compulsivity," and "involuntary." The implication is that there must be an understanding of what is and is not involuntary that makes addiction automatically an involuntary state. In support of this point, the guiding argument in favor of the disease model today is the same as it was in the seventeenth century, despite the advances in scientific understanding. Today, as in the seventeenth century, it is assumed that individuals do not repeatedly engage in self-destructive behavior unless they are compelled to do so. Addiction is a pattern of persistent self-destructive behavior, hence it is involuntary, and as diseases are involuntary, then addiction is a disease. This is perfectly logical, given the assumption that voluntary behavior is necessarily not self-destructive. Again, the issue of whether addiction is a disease depends on the understanding of voluntary behavior.

Can Behavior Be Self-Destructive and Voluntary?

The next section of this chapter asks whether voluntary behavior really does preclude self-destructive behavior. This may seem an odd undertaking, since the meaning of a word is how it is used. If scientists, clinicians, and the public say that voluntary behavior is not self-destructive, then that is what "voluntary" means. Word meanings are not like ancient tablets, waiting to be uncovered by spade and shovel. Day-to-day usage sets the standard. This point was nicely captured by Lewis Carroll in an exchange between Alice and Humpty Dumpty:

> "But 'glory' doesn't mean 'a nice knock-down argument,'" Alice objected.
>
> "When *I* use the word," Humpty Dumpty said, in rather a scornful tone, "it means just what I choose it to mean—neither more nor less."
>
> "The question is," said Alice, "whether you *can* make words mean so many different things."
>
> "The question is," said Humpty Dumpty, "which is to be master—that's all." (Carroll, *Through the Looking-Glass*, p. 102)

But Humpty Dumpty has overlooked something important. How people speak and write is not set in stone. Experience (e.g., new information or a coherent argument) can modify expression, thought, and word usage. As a result, new words emerge and the meanings of old words change. Heat is no longer a "liquid," and of course a whale is no longer a "fish." These changes came about because they made more sense. Possibly, then, it would also be useful to reconsider the definitions of "voluntary" and of "addiction." If "voluntary" is defined in ways that do not preclude self-destructive behavior, then addiction is not automatically a disease. Note that the issue here is not how to identify individuals who use drugs in self-destructive ways. The *DSM* criteria do an excellent job of this. The issue is how to interpret the symptoms. Also, it should be pointed out that coming to a new understanding of the meaning of the terms "voluntary" and "addiction" will not in itself render the problem of addictive drug use any less severe or the plight of the addict any easier. However, it could lead to better treatments, better policy, and better science.

Western culture offers two contradictory visions of voluntary behavior. The seventeenth-century preachers and twenty-first-century addiction scientists take the widely held position that choices are fundamentally rational, hence no one willingly engages in self-destructive acts. This has been formalized in economics, where the assumption is that choices do not simply avoid self-harm but maximize benefits and minimize costs. In contrast to this view, the arts often portray individuals as knowingly, willingly, and persistently pursuing self-destructive ends.

Starting with Homer, self-destructive voluntary behavior makes up much of the content of imaginative literature. In the *Iliad* Agamemnon and Achilles are ruled as much by pride as by reason, and as a result they repeatedly undermine their own interests and those of their followers. According to Homer this is human nature. Millennia later, Philip Roth (2007) records the adventures of an old man, Nathan Zuckerman, who knowingly endangers his well-being for a young woman he can't possibly possess. Zuckerman is 71 years old, suffers from impotence and incontinence, and wears a protective diaper under his pants. He knows that he is being unreasonable but pursues her anyway.

It is hard to argue that Agamemnon and Zuckerman were involuntarily seeking their respective versions of glory. Rather, they plotted their self-made disasters with full awareness of the risks they were taking. It is also hard to argue that these stories do not capture truths about human nature, given that they have been told again and again and listened to avidly for thousands of years. One of the lessons of literature, then (and, I would argue, everyday experience as well), is that voluntary acts are often self-destructive. This implies that self-destructive drug use is not the proper criterion for determining that someone is compulsively using drugs. Likewise, it implies that rationality is not the correct criterion for distinguishing between voluntary and involuntary acts. We need some other approach.

Laboratory studies reveal two types of behavior (e.g., Brown & Herrnstein, 1975; Skinner, 1938). Some actions are elicited by their setting, and others are governed by their consequences. Simple reflexes, instinctive activities, and tics are representative of the first category. Learned behaviors are representative of the second category. To a first approximation, these categories correspond to the labels "involuntary" and "voluntary." For instance, tics are elicited by stimulus conditions and are not reined in by their consequences. In contrast, voluntary actions rise and fall in concert with their benefits and costs. Of course, many behaviors involve a mix of both elicited and learned components. For example, ethologists have shown that "instincts" and "reflexes" involve some learning (e.g., Hailman, 1969), and ritualized compulsions and even tics provide rewards (e.g., the relief of anxiety or release from the pressure that one has to do something). Nevertheless, the distinction between elicited behaviors and consequence-driven behaviors is clear enough to be useful. First, the distinction between the two types of activities will be outlined in more detail, using an example that will be familiar to all readers, and then the rule for distinguishing between elicited and consequence-driven behaviors will be used to evaluate drug use in addicts.

Blinks are involuntary and winks are voluntary. To see why this is so, consider the following similarities and differences. Both have biologies, both are mediated by the brain, both involve facial muscles, and they certainly look similar. Nevertheless, they occur under very different conditions. Winks vary as a function of their consequences, particularly socially mediated ones, whereas blinks are elicited by stimuli and are relatively if not totally immune to their consequences. Readers can prove this for themselves. Have a friend clap her hands loudly near your eyes, but behind your head and unpredictably. You will blink. Now consider the following bet: You get $100 if you successfully suppress the blink but pay $10 to your friend if you blink. Assuming you don't take the bet, imagine that your friend increases the stakes in your favor, so that you get $1000 or even $1,000,000 for not blinking. The added incentives will fail to increase the likelihood of "not blinking," assuming the experiment is done with unpredictable and loud claps. This is because blinks are "wired up" so that they are free of the influence of brain structures that mediate the motivational effects of costs and benefits. This has its advantages. When it comes to the defense of something as vital as the eyes, fast, automatic, stimulus-driven responses are needed—not mulling over. Now consider winks.

It is my impression that for the last twenty years or so winks, particularly the male-to-female type, have been on the wane. They seem relics of an era of hidden sex and may even be sexist. In any case, everyday experience suggests that winks would all but disappear under the least social pressure. Just the threat of embarrassment would persuade a "habitual" winker to cease. Note that the distinction between winks and blinks is not one of free will versus determinism. Rather, the difference resides in the underlying neural controls. For example, neuropsychological studies show that voluntary and involuntary facial responses have different underlying neural circuits. Reflexive facial actions are under the control of lower brain areas and pyramidal nerves. Voluntary facial actions are under the control of the cortical motor strip and extra-pyramidal nerve fibers (e.g., Rinn, 1984).

These contrasts provide a rule for determining whether an activity is voluntary or involuntary. Voluntary activities vary as a function of costs, benefits, the opinions of others, cultural values, and the myriad of other factors that influence decisions. Involuntary activities vary little or not at all as a function of the factors that influence decisions. Thus, we can test whether drug use in addicts is voluntary by testing whether it is brought to a halt by the factors that influence decisions. Some of this evidence has already been presented. But before reviewing the findings, there is a practical side to the matter of what is voluntary that requires comment.

It may not always be feasible to apply sufficiently powerful consequences. Hunger and eating provide a familiar example. Eating is voluntary. Although food is essential, successful hunger strikes show that individuals can be persuaded not to eat. But the motivational strength of hunger plus the fact that calories have no substitutes say that for most people a contingency that rewarded not-eating would soon fail. Similarly, contingencies that have the more limited aim of reducing eating do not fare well for the same reasons. The issue is not that food seeking is really a reflex (although digestion is), it is that there are no legitimate or practical alternatives to food. Thus, the definition of what is voluntary should be expanded to include feasibility. We can say, then, that the degree to which an activity is voluntary is the degree to which it systematically varies as a function of its consequences, and the degree to which it is feasible to apply such consequences.

Western culture offers two opposing views as to whether voluntary behavior can be persistently self-destructive. According to the view that an individual cannot willingly and persistently engage in self-harm, addiction is necessarily compulsive drug use because addiction is also self-destructive drug use. The corollary of this position is that addiction must be a disease. Seventeenth-century preachers and the addiction researchers cited above staked out this position. The idea that voluntary behavior can be self-destructive implies that addiction is not necessarily a compulsive, involuntary state. To determine which account is correct, we need a definition of voluntariness that is silent about rationality. The idea that behaviors can be evaluated in terms of the degree to which they vary as a function of their consequences does just this. According to this rule, voluntary activities vary systematically as a function of their consequences, where the consequences include benefits, costs, and values. In contrast, involuntary activities are elicited by preceding stimuli (e.g., urges) and are influenced little or not at all by their consequences. This difference reflects differences in the neural connections that link the activity to its consequences, which is to say, the issue is not free will. It was also pointed out that there was an issue of feasibility. If there are no legitimate or practical contingencies available, then the activity is functionally involuntary. With this background it is now possible to test whether drug use in addicts is voluntary. If the factors that affect everyday decisions are the same as those that affect drug use in addicts, it is voluntary. However, if the scale of these factors is such that they are not legitimate—say, only the threat of severe punishment brings drug use to a halt in addicts— then for practical purposes, drug use in addicts is involuntary.

Some of the relevant findings for this exercise have already been presented. According to the self-reports presented in Chapter 3, financial concerns, fear of arrest, and values regarding parenthood brought drug use to a halt in addicts. According to the surveys presented in Chapter 4, most addicts quit by their early thirties, and most of those who quit did so outside of the purview of treatment clinics. This suggests that the everyday business of life, particularly the changes that accompany adulthood such as financial and family pressures, motivated addicts to stop using drugs. However, both lines of evidence fail to meet the threshold of scientific proof. Self-reports are not replicable, and the explanation of why most addicts quit is inferential. What is needed is an experimental procedure that captures the essence of the self-reports and inferences regarding the influence of everyday pressures on drug use. The study presented next meets these criteria.

Will Modest, Everyday Incentives Stop Drug Use in Addicts?

Chapter 4 ended with the description of a number of treatment programs that successfully reduced drug use. They shared three features. The drug users were doctors or airplane pilots; they were tested randomly for drug use; and if they tested positive for drugs they could lose their jobs and professional careers. The follow-up studies reported abstinence rates of 85 percent or more. However, these are severe consequences, and the contingency is probably not a practical one for most clinics and most addicts. It is unlikely that programs that threatened job loss would win broad public support, and a good proportion of those with drug problems may already be unemployed. Thus, it would be useful to test whether contingencies work when the stakes are not so great.

Earning vouchers through drug-free metabolic tests. Steve Higgins, a psychologist at the University of Vermont, developed an addiction treatment program based on the idea that immediate and concrete but modest incentives could persuade addicts to quit using drugs. His initial target population was cocaine addicts (Higgins et al., 1991). This is significant because at the time of the initial study (the late 1980s), it was widely believed that cocaine addiction was intractable. There were no pharmacological treatments, and clinicians reported that relapse was the norm.

The Vermont clinic pursued a two-pronged anti-drug strategy. First, there were counseling sessions that helped the patients develop a new, drug-free life style. The focus was on practical matters such as how to find a better job, how to establish better relations with family members, and how to obtain training that promised a brighter future. Second, there was an exchange system that offered vouchers for metabolic evidence of drug abstinence. The patients were tested several times a week for drug use. If the tests were negative, they earned vouchers that could be traded in for desirable but modest goods, such as sports equipment and movie passes. The contingency also gave a bonus for continuously maintaining abstinence. Each additional week of abstinence increased the value of the voucher. Conversely, a urine test that revealed evidence of drug use set the value of the voucher back to its initial, lowest level. Thus, abstinence earned immediate rewards that introduced or strengthened activities that had the potential to compete with drug use, and consistency increased the value of the contingency. There were also two control groups to help identify which features of the program were essential to its success. Some patients received traditional psychological counseling and some received vouchers independent of whether they had been abstinent.

Over a series of tests, the contingency groups always had higher abstinence rates (e.g., Higgins et al., 1991, 1994, 1995). For instance, in one of the early cocaine experiments, about 70 percent of the voucher subjects were continuously drug-free for the first five weeks of the program, whereas fewer than 20 percent of the patients in traditional counseling maintained abstinence for the first five weeks (Higgins et al., 1994). Although the success rates were much greater than expected given the belief that addiction is a chronic, relapsing disease, the success rates were not as high as in the doctor/pilot programs. Presumably this was because the stakes were lower. Careers were not on the line, and the dollar value of the vouchers did not exceed twelve dollars a day. Even discounting for the Vermont economy, this is a fraction of the losses that the physicians and pilots faced. Indeed, the vouchers were probably worth less money than the subjects had been spending on cocaine. Yet, most of the treatment subjects preferred vouchers to cocaine, their addiction notwithstanding.

On most occasions, most of the subjects in the behavioral program were willing to give up cocaine for vouchers worth between $2.50 and $12 a day. But what would happen once the contingency was removed? If the contract's influence was strictly of the moment, then once the clinic closed its doors, the "addicts" would sell the goods they had obtained with vouchers to buy cocaine. But if the contingencies and counseling led to new activities, new hobbies, or better relationships with family members, then the newly acquired interests might squeeze out drug use just as drug use had squeezed out competing activities prior to treatment.

Do the changes in drug use last? A subsequent study addressed whether the subjects would relapse once the contingency was removed (e.g., Higgins et al., 2000). As before there was a voucher group and also a control group receiving traditional counseling. The voucher group earned various prosocial rewards for drug-free urine tests and participated in counseling programs that promoted rewarding, drug-free activities. The control group received traditional drug counseling. Figure 5.2 shows the results.

The darker bars show the contingency/voucher subjects. At every follow-up date, the voucher subjects were more likely to remain drug-free, even though the contingency was no longer in effect. Moreover, at every follow-up test, the percentage of drug-free voucher subjects increased, rising from about 60 to almost 80 percent over the year. The post-treatment increase suggests that the contingency set in motion positive, self-sustaining behavioral patterns. Just as heavy drug use initiates a downward spiral of increasingly negative consequences and decreasing options, healthy alternative activities can set in motion an upward spiral of increasingly positive consequences and increasing options.

There are other choice-based treatment programs, and like the one at the University of Vermont, they too have had some success. For instance,

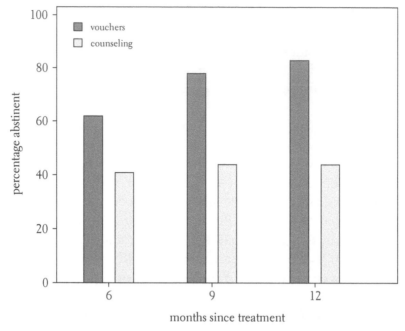

5.2 Post-treatment abstinence for cocaine addicts. The abstinence rate for those in the voucher program increased over time (even though the contingency was no longer in effect). Data from Higgins et al., 2000.

a recent review concluded that contingency management is "one of the most effective" treatments for chemical dependencies (Prendergast et al., 2006).

Are We Free to Choose Addiction?

In the introduction to this chapter, it was pointed out that the disease interpretation has been justified in terms of its clinical benefits, the fact that addiction has a biological basis, and the assertion that addicts are involuntary drug users. There is a fourth justification that is not usually discussed but has probably played an important role in thinking about addiction. This is the idea that addiction is a disease because addicts do not make "free" choices but determined choices. In a paper titled "Comparison of alcoholism and other medical diseases: An internist's view," Dr. David Lewis (1991) says this idea has played a "paramount" role in classifying diseases: "If the etiology and/or course of the disease appears to be primarily under the control of an individual, then it is thought to be a moral problem. If, on the other hand, the etiology and/or course of the condition is primarily beyond the control or intention of the individual, it is more acceptable to call that condition a disease."

Lewis is not, it seems, defending this view but making an observation regarding how people think about the causes of human behavior and the implications of these ideas for classifying disorders. The view is problematic when applied to voluntary behavior. As science has learned more about behavior, it has become increasingly clear that the causes that matter are often well beyond anyone's control. We have learned that factors such as as genes, hormones, neurotransmitters, cohort, and gender play a large role in voluntary behavior. Now couple the scientific findings with the assumption that human disorders are subject to two different types of causal relations: those that one is able to control and those that one cannot control. The implication is that as we learn more about a disorder, the more likely it is to be thought of as a disease. For instance, as we learn more, the causes become more remote, and if they are remote, then they are not under one's control, and hence the disorder can be classified as a disease. Lewis's observations help explain why support for the disease interpretation has increased over time. They predict that as other behavioral disorders are better understood, the tendency to think of them as diseases will also increase. Put more generally, the idea that there are causes under one's control and causes beyond one's control ends up defining voluntary behavior as behavior that is not understood.

Craving and Voluntary Behavior

One of the characteristics of heavy drug use is craving. A search in the Internet resource database PsycInfo for "craving" and ("addiction" or "dependence") yields almost eighteen hundred different references; the third edition of the *DSM* listed "craving" as a symptom of dependence; and many researchers and clinicians explain addiction as a function of craving, particularly if they assume that addiction means compulsive drug use. For example, in a recent article that appeared in the journal *Addiction*, the authors write that craving is "a psychological state characterized by obsessive thoughts and compulsive behaviour" (Hillemacher et al., 2006). The idea is that cravings are "irresistible urges" that trigger bouts of compulsive drug use. However, craving has proven a controversial term. It was dropped from the list of symptoms in later editions of the *DSM*, and many researchers have pointed out that the term is often used without much heed to how to best measure it, which is a way of saying that its referents are not clear or the authors' intended meaning is not supported by the data (e.g., Kozlowski & Wilkinson, 1987). Nevertheless, "craving" holds a special place in drug research, and as such it deserves attention.

Craving has seen most service as an explanation of relapse. The idea is that even if someone has vowed to quit and has taken serious measures to do so, he or she is not able to prevent cravings, and the cravings trigger drug use. Thus, cravings invade consciousness and because of their intensity overwhelm even the most sincere intentions. The strong version of this account is that cravings make drug use inevitable. More tempered accounts predict that cravings increase during abstinence and that cravings increase the likelihood of relapse, although not to the point of insuring relapse. Chapters 3 and 4 provide results that are relevant to the strong version of craving's role in addiction.

Patty and Jessie (Chapter 3) volunteered that they experienced cravings for cocaine but found ways of resisting them. Their experience has to be rather typical. If most addicts quit and cravings are common, then millions of addicts must have experienced cravings to resume drug use but learned how not to give in to them. Thus, cravings are not a sufficient condition for drug use; they do not make it obligatory.

Although cravings do not trigger compulsive drug use, cravings may increase the likelihood of drug use, and if cravings increased during abstinence, they would pose a major threat to quitting. A particularly thorough study addresses both issues. Saul Shiffman and his colleagues at the University of Pittsburgh and Carnegie Mellon University (1997) measured the relationship between craving and the relapse in 214 volunteer subjects who had recently quit smoking. The subjects reported on cravings four to five times a day at random intervals and in the morning when the urge to smoke is typically greatest. They were asked to estimate the strength of their urge to smoke, whether they had smoked, and the circumstances surrounding temptations to smoke. This study went on for about a month, resulting in tens of thousands of data points and what is correctly called a natural history of craving and relapse.

Craving decreased with the onset of abstinence. The authors point out that this result is surprising given the role that craving has played in addiction theory, but that a decrease in craving with abstinence may not actually be so surprising in light of other findings. This point will be returned to. Although craving decreased, it was not unrelated to relapse.

The strength of the urge to smoke upon waking predicted the resumption of smoking. But, curiously, the strength of urges during the day that were closer in time to the actual lapse did not predict smoking. Other researchers have replicated the Pittsburgh study results, finding that there is typically a relationship between global measures of craving, for example, those taken during the first week or so of abstinence, and later relapse (e.g., Bottlender & Soyka, 2004; Killen & Fortmann, 1997). And it also should be pointed out that for current drug users there is a positive correlation between urges to use drugs and drug use (e.g., Shiffman et al., 2002).

Cravings, then, are one of the factors that influence drug use. An urge is not an obligation, and as the biographies and other studies show, drug users vary in how they respond to urges. Most drug users quit, so most drug users end up, like Patty and Jessie, finding alternatives to drugs when cravings enter consciousness.

But what determines whether cravings enter consciousness? The conventional account is that they are conditioned, as in associative learning. However, the finding that cravings decreased at the onset of abstinence suggests that there is more to the etiology of craving than associative learning. It is uncomfortable to crave something that you cannot have, whereas craving something that you will get for sure may add to its enjoyment. This suggests that the joy of savoring future pleasure may increase cravings, whereas the discomfort at knowing that a desired event will not occur may decrease craving. The data fit this interpretation. When drug cues, such as cigarettes and a lighter, predicted that there would not be an opportunity to use the drug, drug cravings decreased, but when the same cues predicted a strong or sure chance to use the drug, drug cravings increased (e.g., Carter & Tiffany, 2001; Dols et al., 2000; Meyer & Mirin, 1979). This helps explain why drug users typically report that their urges decline as abstinence continues, and it also suggests that there is an instrumental component to urges. In the experiments there is a correlation between the frequency of urges and their consequences. What remains to be established is whether this correlation reflects a causal connection between urges and their consequences.

Thus, craving fits into the general framework of this book. Cravings do not trigger bouts of compulsive drug use, and they do not make drug use obligatory. Rather, they are one of the several factors that influence drug use. In addition, biographical accounts and experiments suggest that urges themselves vary as a function of their consequences, which means that to some extent they may include a voluntary component.

Summary

According to the research results reviewed in Chapters 2, 3, and 4, most addicts choose to stop using drugs by about age thirty, and the reasons that they do so are by and large the same as the reasons that motivate most of our actions, such as finances, job, family responsibilities, and self-esteem. The conceptual analysis presented in this chapter revealed that the idea that addiction is a disease has been based on a limited view of voluntary behavior. In these accounts the influence of genes or even antecedents that were beyond an individual's control implied that an activity was not voluntary. These limitations do not square with the facts. Genes and factors that are "beyond one's control" influence activities that everyone agrees are voluntary, such as participation in religion and cohort-specific activities. Nevertheless, the fact that word usage defines word meaning says it is perfectly legitimate to proceed as if self-destructive drug use implied involuntary drug use. Legitimacy is not the same as coherence, however, and the idea that addiction is compulsive ends up being incoherent. For instance, we saw that individuals who have been using heroin on a daily basis for years decided to quit and then did so (e.g., Scott in Chapter 3). If we held to the view that addiction was compulsive drug use, we would have to say that "Scott decided not to compulsively take heroin every day when he figured out that he could no longer afford it." Or, in light of the epidemiological findings, we would have to say, "Most people who are compulsive drug users spontaneously decide to quit as they enter adulthood." These sentences do violence to the English language.

There is, though, a way to speak sensibly about addiction. Research reveals two categories of behavior: activities that are elicited by antecedent states and activities that are governed by consequences that were experienced in the past and are anticipated. This is a useful distinction because we can then test if voluntary implies rationality rather than assume this to be the case. Since drug use in addicts is governed by its consequences, the answer is that voluntary is not necessarily rational. This, I would argue, we already knew. The subject matter of heroic tales and novels is voluntary behavior, and a recurring story line is the man or woman who knowingly pursues ends that bring about great suffering to himself or herself and others. In any case, given the distinction between voluntary and elicited behavior, it is possible to talk coherently about addiction. Voluntary behavior has a biological basis; addiction has a biological basis. Voluntary acts are guided by costs and benefits, such as concern about family, cultural values, self-esteem, fear of punishment, and so on; the same holds for drug use in addicts. Thus, it is possible to talk coherently about addiction if voluntary behavior is defined as that subset of acts that are susceptible to the influence of their consequences.

There are additional advantages to the approach to voluntary action described here. It is supported by the vision of human behavior in imaginative literature and it is in accord with informal social practices as well as legislation. If rationality is the criterion for voluntary action, then we would have to conclude that works of fiction are really clinical case studies rather than explorations of human nature under varying circumstances. My view is that the latter interpretation makes more sense. In a quite different realm, we can see the research-based understanding of voluntary and involuntary behavior in conventional attitudes. Society treats sneezing and spitting as qualitatively different behaviors. Sneezing is treated as symptomatic of a disease; spitting is treated as symptomatic of bad manners. These differences in turn reflect the fact that rewards and punishments have much more of an influence on spitting than sneezing. Even though sneezing is more likely to spread disease, we regulate spitting.

This example leads to the legislative version of the distinction between voluntary and involuntary acts. Judicial systems distinguish between acts that are subject to punishment and those that are not. This distinction is sometimes explained in terms of free will and responsibility. Individuals are responsible for acts that they freely choose and should not be blamed for ones that are compelled. However, I believe that an examination of how the distinction actually works will reveal that according to Western legal traditions, individuals are usually held responsible for those activities that are susceptible to the influence of their consequences and, conversely, individuals are not responsible for those activities that vary little or not at all as a function of consequences. For example, Patty Hearst said she robbed a bank because she was forced to do so upon threat of death by her kidnappers. Willie Sutton is famous for saying he robbed banks because "that's where the money is." If Patty Hearst was telling the truth, then we should distinguish her case from Willie Sutton's. It is unreasonable to expect legally mediated consequences to trump the immediate threat of death. In contrast, Willie Sutton had alternatives, which means that legally mediated consequences could have some effect. (Patty Hearst's testimony was not considered believable by many, but she did get a reduced sentence.)

Although there are many sources of support for the vision of voluntary behavior that has been presented in this chapter, it is incomplete. There is no explanation of how behavior can be both voluntary and self-destructive. To be sure, the empirical and logical relations introduced in this and previous chapters support the statement that "addicts voluntarily choose to use drugs in a self-destructive manner." But nothing has been said as to how this comes about. Theories of motivation and choice typically predict good if not optimal outcomes. Thus, the conclusion that addiction is self-destructive yet voluntary calls for an explanation.

The facts and logic presented in this chapter do not say that it is always the case that someone addicted to drugs can choose to quit. Voluntary behavior is not the same as free will. Many addicts have limitations (for example, medical problems) that make it difficult to take advantage of alternatives to drugs, and for many addicts there are road blocks that prevent assistance from agencies that could intervene on their behalf. As described in the next chapter, under certain conditions the immediate costs of quitting are greater than the immediate benefits of quitting. In this situation, only a change in the setting can lead to a decrease in drug use. The "intervention" has to lead to changes in how the drug user approaches his or her alternatives, or else it must affect the values of the alternatives themselves. Thus, the conclusion that addiction involves voluntary drug use does not imply that quitting will be easy, and in some situations it says that it may be impossible.

6

ADDICTION AND CHOICE

The Great Lisbon Earthquake of 1755 was described by church officials as a sign that God was unhappy with the sinful behavior of the residents of that city. Voltaire and other Enlightenment intellectuals saw this great earthquake as evidence that nature was not guided by reason. More recently, fundamentalist Internet sites interpreted Hurricane Katrina as a call to the "sin-loving and rebellious" citizens of New Orleans and environs to repent. The church and Enlightenment interpretations of the Lisbon earthquake were consonant with their times. Both views assume that a grand purpose guides nature, whereas today supernatural explanations for Katrina seem anachronistic to most. Newspapers and school curricula explain hurricanes in terms of impersonal, physical forces, in which neither God nor reason plays a role. What the science-based accounts reveal is that extreme environmental events do not imply supernatural causes or even special principles. The physics of heat exchange, air pressure, moisture, and wind explain the modest and familiar transitions from a warm, quiet afternoon to a cool, breezy evening as well as the tumultuous and less common transitions from a tropical depression to the devastatingly high winds and drenching rains of a hurricane. The different outcomes reflect differences in the prevailing conditions, such as differences in latitude and water temperature, but not differences in governing principles.

Just as the diurnal cool breezes at evening and the once-in-a-lifetime hurricane are explained by the same physical principles, so in this chapter everyday choices and addiction will be explained by the same motivational principles. The motivational principles are simple and self-evident. Under ordinary conditions, they combine to produce adaptive if not optimal choices. But when one of the options is an addictive drug, these same principles can lead to addiction. If we were to choose among conventional items, say groceries and clothing, the ones that were most preferred would most likely also be beneficial and possibly even optimal as measured by long-term economic criteria. But if one of the options is an addictive drug, the principles that resulted in a smooth-running household would now lead to excessive drug use, a decrease in overall welfare, and regret. Hurricanes depend on general physical principles and a unique set of events that become more likely in tropical latitudes in the early fall. Addiction depends on general principles of choice, the unique behavioral effects of addictive drugs, and individual and environmental factors that affect decision making. Hurricanes and addiction are out of the ordinary and disastrous, yet they reflect general rather than special principles.

Voluntary behavior is a huge, sprawling topic. Most human activity involves learned actions that are not elicited but are contingent on circumstances and history. Although reflexes and instincts play a critical role in human behavior, particularly among newborns, in dynamic environments, such as the surface of Earth, humans and other living creatures depend largely on actions that are shaped more by experience than by DNA. For humans, virtually all environments support more than one activity, so that in effect most behavior is choice behavior. Indeed most of what all mammals do most of the time is voluntary. Consequently, it is not practical to introduce the topic of voluntary behavior by reviewing its literature. Instead, I will use a single representative case. The case is hypothetical but serves the purpose of introducing principles that apply to actual voluntary activities. It is based on one introduced by Richard Herrnstein (1990b), and I have used it to introduce the study of choice to my students.

> Imagine that for the foreseeable future you will eat out every night at either a Chinese or an Italian restaurant. Tell me how you would decide which one to eat at. The following conditions hold. (1) Prior to eating in either restaurant, your initial preference is for Chinese food. However, your preferences change as a function of which restaurant you choose. (2) Eating one type of food reduces your preference for it due to habituation. Conversely, not eating the other type of food increases your preference for it because of dishabituation. (3) The habituation and dishabituation processes are stronger for Chinese than for Italian. That is, your taste for Chinese sours more

quickly, but also regains its lost value more quickly. Tell me
how you would proceed.

After repeating this description, I then ask the audience how they
would choose a restaurant. The responses are surprisingly uniform. Almost everyone says that each night they would go to the restaurant that
they currently preferred. Given the description, they say that this would
usually be Chinese, but not always. Sometimes they would eat at the Italian restaurant, but then they would switch back to Chinese, and so on.

Although this approach seems sensible, if not ideal—what could be
better than always doing what you liked best? there are usually a few
people who offer a different approach. In so many words, they suggest
that because the meals change in value as a function of which one was
chosen, it might be better to let the favorite type of meal get really good
and then choose it. Implicit in this strategy is the idea that there might be
an advantage in avoiding the option that is the current favorite.

The two strategies are similar in that the governing principle is to
choose what is best. However, they differ in how they define the options, and this proves important. In the first and more likely strategy, the
restaurant-goer evaluated each restaurant in terms of its value at the moment of choice. The issue was which restaurant was best tonight. Although it was pointed out that meals changed in value as a function of
how frequently they were chosen, the manner in which tonight's meal influenced the value of future meals was not part of the calculation. What
mattered were the current values of the two cuisines. In contrast, the idea
of letting the value of the Chinese restaurant increase implies that the
choice involves more than the current values of the competing options.
The build-up takes time, so that each option is necessarily a series of
meals. Moreover, in order to let the Chinese meal get better, the series of
meals will have to contain some Italian meals, and there will be days in
which it will be necessary to consume a less-desirable Italian meal in order to have a really great Chinese meal in the future. That is, there is the
possibility of a conflict between the choice dictated by the day-by-day
strategy and the choice dictated by the multiple-day strategy. Thus, the
hypothetical restaurant problem yields two patterns of making choices.
Most respondents consider the issue as simply one of choosing which restaurant is best at the moment of choice. A minority take a different approach; they suggest a strategy that reflects the fact that choices also im-

pact the future values of the meals and the overall value of eating out. They, in effect, redefine the options as competing meal plans. In one case the options are single items; in the other case the options are aggregates composed of the single items.

The pattern of responses to the restaurant problem has been very predictable. I can count on most people agreeing with the one-meal-at-a-time, current-value approach, and then, perhaps with a bit of coaxing, others proposing the more complex, multimeal approach. The most interesting aspect of the demonstration, though, is what it reveals about voluntary behavior. The responses can be restated as three principles. These principles are simple, prove to be quite general, and are self-evident. But when they are combined, they generate predictions that are not at all self-evident. The predictions range from optimal choices to suboptimal choices, including patterns of behavior that approximate those associated with addiction and even drug binging. That is, the responses to the restaurant problem serve as the input for a set of ideas that helps explain addiction as well as everyday choices. In keeping with the natural disaster example that began this chapter, the principles will be applied to ordinary "commodities" as well as to drugs. If the analogy with the physical world holds, the predictions should generate a familiar and reasonable pattern of behavior when the choice items are the ordinary items of everyday life, but a destructive pattern of behavior when one of the choices is an addictive drug.

Preferences are dynamic. In the restaurant problem, choices and value were mutually dependent. Eating Chinese food reduced its future value and increased the future value of Italian food, and vice versa for eating Italian food. This pattern is typical. New activities are exciting at first but then become boring; sports are fun but then get tiring; after a few hours of reading, our eyes get tired, and so on. The dynamic interactions can be quite complex, with values shifting both up and down. Potato chips and other salty foods become tastier at first, but as eating proceeds, they eventually lose their allure and can even become aversive. Similar dynamics hold for sweet foods. It is harder to stop eating chocolate after a few bites than it is to refrain from eating chocolate altogether. For some commodities, value can take an ever-increasing trajectory. People who are in "love" with skilled activities, such as piano playing, or a field of study, say literature, find ever-increasing enjoyment as they become more skilled and more knowledgeable. But, regardless of the particulars, choice and value interact dynamically. Individuals make choices based on the values of the outcomes, and, in turn, the choices alter the values of the outcomes.

Given a series of choices, there is more than one way to frame the possible options. It is always possible to choose between the available items one at a time, or to organize the items into sequences and then choose between different sequences. This will be called local and global choice. Deciding each night which meal is better is the local approach. Deciding between sequences composed of both Chinese and Italian meals is the global approach. Local choice is simple, but it ignores the dynamics that link choice and changes in value. In global choice, the options (meal sequences) reflect the dynamic relationships between choice and changes in value.

Individuals always choose the better option. In local choice, choosing the better option means choosing the item that currently has the higher value. In global choice, the best choice is the collection or sequence of items that has higher value. The local-choice approach is also called "melioration" and has been the focus of a series of highly influential empirical and theoretical studies (e.g., Herrnstein & Prelec, 1992; Vaughan, 1981).

These three principles summarize the responses to the restaurant problem. To see what they imply for the understanding of voluntary behavior, I have put together a series of graphs that apply these principles to different commodities, including drugs. The first graph, Figure 6.1, shows the implications for the restaurant problem. This example provides some sense of what the principles imply for typical, everyday choices. The figure charts the choices of a pair of restaurant-goers. As in the hypothetical problem, they initially liked Chinese food more than Italian food. Their preferences changed as a function of choice, and one restaurant-goer framed his options locally (top panel), and the other framed his options globally (bottom panel). Importantly, the initial meal values and rate at which meals changed in value as a function of choice were the same in both panels. This was insured by using equations to generate the graphs. These equations specified the values of Chinese and Italian meals as a function of the number of times each restaurant had been selected in the

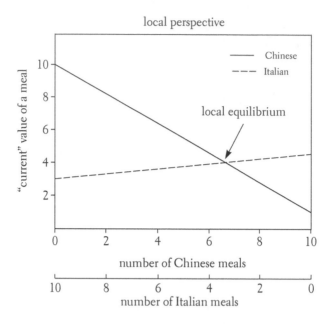

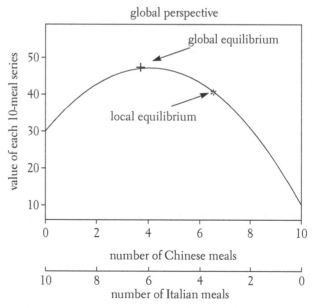

6.1 The hypothetical restaurant problem. Although the situation is dynamic (i.e., value changes as a function of choice), choice proportions stabilize for both the local frame of reference (top panel) and the global frame of reference. However, as shown in the bottom panel, global choice earns more.

just-previous ten meals, and for each panel the equations are the same.[1] However, in the top panel the equations were arranged so that they show the current value of each cuisine, whereas in the bottom panel the equations were combined so that they show the values of every possible combination of ten meals.[2] That is, the equations reflect the difference between local choice and global choice.

These different ways of framing the options (and arranging the equations) can be described in terms of the inner dialog that might accompany the decision-making process. For the hypothetical person represented by the top panel, the conversation might go something like, "I think I would like to eat Chinese food tonight; it is almost always my favorite." For the bottom panel, the conversation is likely to be something like, "I find that dining out is more pleasurable when I don't always go to my favorite restaurant. I save it for when I really want a great meal. Eating out is most enjoyable when I space my meals better." Each approach yields a predictable outcome, but they prove to be different. Also, it should be pointed out that the graphs include the assumption that each meal has the same price, so that they differ only in terms of how much enjoyment they provide.

The hypothetical person who took the meal-at-a-time approach ends up at a stable overall choice proportion, which is the point at which the two lines cross (see note 2 for details). This will be called the "local equilibrium." At the local equilibrium, the current values of the two meals are the same. As a result, after a few Chinese meals, the Italian cuisine will now appear to be the better choice. Similarly, after one or two Italian meals, the Chinese restaurant will now appear to be the better choice. Thus, a stable overall choice proportion emerges even though the values of the meals continue to change as a function of choice.

The hypothetical person who framed the problem as one of finding the best meal plan also ends up at a stable overall choice proportion. This is the point at which the curve showing the value of each possible meal plan attains its maximum value. This will be called the "global equilibrium." This choice proportion is stable because there is no better way of allocating choices. If the distribution of meals began to stray from the best meal plan, enjoyment would decrease, and this would motivate a realignment back to the combination that produced the peak eating experience. Thus, a restaurant-goer who pictures eating out in terms of the best combination of meals will always end up at the global equilibrium.

Figure 6.1 reveals a surprising result. Even though the graphs were set up so that the values of the restaurants were exactly the same and the habituation and dishabituation rates were exactly the same, the two ways of framing the options led to a different pattern of choices. The local equilibrium stabilized at approximately seven (6.7) Chinese meals for every three Italian meals, so that there was an overall preference for Chinese food. The global equilibrium stabilized at four Chinese meals for every six Italian meals, so that there was an overall preference for Italian food. The difference is not neutral. The hypothetical person who framed the problem as one of competing meal plans gained about 20 percent more enjoyment from eating out than the local bookkeeping, current-value restaurant-goer. This increment in overall dining-out pleasure did not require any extra response costs in terms of number of meals. Rather, it was obtained by avoiding the Chinese meal on days that it would afford more pleasure than an Italian meal, so that its value would increase even more. This may exact a psychological cost and the plan itself may exact cognitive costs, but in terms of physical effort or monetary expense (recall, it is assumed that all meals have the same price), the two approaches are identical. Thus, how the options were framed made a difference, all else being the same.

The Lessons of Dining Out

If the principles that generated Figure 6.1 commonly apply—and not just to eating out—then the local equilibrium and global equilibrium should predict patterns of behavior observed in research studies. This proves to be the case. The local equilibrium is equivalent to one of the most robust empirical results in the study of choice. In laboratory and natural settings, choice proportions approximate ("match") reward proportions. This is called the "matching law" (Herrnstein, 1970), and it is the same as the local equilibrium (e.g., Vaughan, 1981). As suggested by the label "matching law," matching (the local equilibrium) occurs over a wide range of conditions. The subjects have included humans, pigeons, rats, cows, monkeys, and opossums; that is, every species which has been studied to date. The rewards have included items that can be consumed, such as food and water, the opportunity to run in a wheel, money, and signs of social approval. And the settings have included both conventional laboratory research chambers as well as natural environments (for reviews, see Davison & McCarthy, 1988; Herrnstein, 1997; Williams,

1988). In other words, over a remarkably wide range of conditions, individuals make choices as predicted by the local equilibrium.

Although choices typically gravitate to the local equilibrium, it is possible to arrange conditions so that the distribution of choices approximates the global equilibrium (e.g., Heyman & Tanz, 1995; Kudadjie-Gyamfi & Rachlin, 1996). As suggested by the fact that this result is much less common, special efforts are usually required to insure the effect. These efforts are described later in this chapter. The global equilibrium is also the result that economics textbooks predict. In chapters on consumer choice, hypothetical shoppers invariably choose between competing "market baskets." The market baskets are examples of the aggregates or series of choices (e.g., "meal plans") that in this chapter are the basic units of global choice. In other words, the conventional economic analysis of choice assumes a global frame of reference. Ignoring bookkeeping costs, consumers should adopt a global frame of reference. Presumably, this is what economic advisors advocate and what businesses who follow economic principles try to do. Thus, there is no shortage of empirical support for the models of choice displayed in Figure 6.1. The local equilibrium approximates the results of hundreds of research studies, and the global equilibrium approximates how economists say choices should be made.

The second major implication of Figure 6.1 is that voluntary behavior does not necessarily lead to the best outcome. In the top panel choice proportions stabilized at a suboptimal equilibrium. This was a logical consequence of the three principles and the fact that the meals had different initial values. This result stands in contrast to most analyses of choice. As just pointed out, in economics it is assumed that choices are guided by the global equilibrium. There is no mention of any other possibility or competing ways to frame the options. Similarly, psychological theories of choice do not describe competing frames of reference, one tied to the local equilibrium and one tied to the global equilibrium. Thus, the restaurant problem suggests that analyses of choice have been too narrow.

The third implication of Figure 6.1 is that voluntary behavior and overconsumption go hand in hand. The way to maximize the experience of eating out was to choose four Chinese meals for every six Italian ones. But the local equilibrium led to about seven Chinese meals for every three Italian ones. From the perspective of global choice, this is almost two times too many Chinese meals. Thus, the hypothetical diner who framed his options from a local perspective ate less well because he ate too much Chinese food. As the local equilibrium approximates what is typically found in both laboratory and natural settings, the message is that some degree of overconsumption usually accompanies voluntary actions.

The fourth implication of Figure 6.1 is psychological. There were two possible outcomes, and each was best from its respective frame of reference. This means that at least some of the time the contingencies that guide voluntary behaviors are ambiguous. For example, for someone who evenly divided his meals between the two restaurants, local-choice bookkeeping says to go to the Chinese restaurant, whereas global-choice bookkeeping says to go to the Italian restaurant. Assuming that the restaurant-goer was aware of these two ways of making choices, he or she would feel ambivalence and possibly regret. Just as there is a viewpoint from which either choice is best, there is also a viewpoint from which either choice is worst. For those who tend to punish themselves, voluntary behavior provides plenty of ammunition.

Figure 6.1 provides a concise summary of key features of literally hundreds of studies on choice. Its implications differ from the understanding of choice that has informed the discussion of addiction. It shows that choice can stabilize at a suboptimal level of benefits, that suboptimal yet voluntary outcomes involve overconsumption of at least one of the options, and that the contingencies that guide choice are ambiguous. These conclusions are at odds with the assumption that voluntary actions are guided by rationality. Indeed they suggest that voluntary action and addiction differ in degree, not kind. For example, relapse and attempts to quit using drugs are signs of ambivalence, addiction by definition means excessive drug use, and to say that addiction is a disorder is to say that it is not an optimal pattern of behavior.

Graphing Addiction

Figure 6.2 tests whether the principles that described choosing a restaurant can generate a graph that models addiction. The *DSM* account of addiction provided the guidelines of how to create the graph. It states that the essential feature of addiction is the continued use of drugs despite "significant substance-related problems." These problems necessarily occur in the course of nondrug activities. For example, withdrawal interferes with doing well at work and intoxication torpedoes conventional

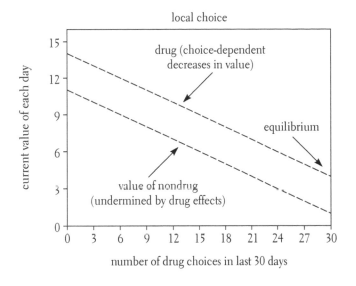

local choice

drug (choice-dependent
decreases in value)

equilibrium

value of nondrug
(undermined by drug effects)

number of drug choices in last 30 days

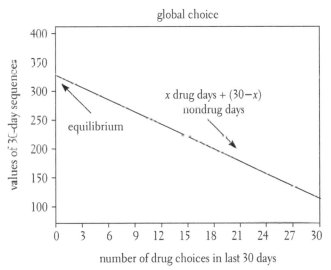

global choice

x drug days + (30−x)
nondrug days

equilibrium

number of drug choices in last 30 days

6.2 Choice for drug and nondrug days, where the properties of the drug mimic those assumed in the *DSM-IV* description of addiction.

interactions. Thus, the graph should show that as drug use increases, the value of the competing nondrug activities decreases. As drugs also lose value as a function of use, as in tolerance, the graph should also show consumption-dependent decreases in value for the drug. Figure 6.2 shows what is probably the simplest possible version of these two properties. As before, the top panel represents local choice, which in this case is the decision to get high or not get high on a day-by-day basis, and the bottom panel shows global choice, which in this case is a decision about the overall number of days of intoxication in thirty-day bundles.

As in Figure 6.1, the equations establish that the initial values of the competing choice items and the manner in which their value changes as a function of choice is the same in both panels. For example, in a day-by-day frame of reference, the two hypothetical drug users like days with drugs better than days without drugs by exactly the same amount, and, similarly, they experience tolerance and dishabituation at exactly the same rates. However, since they frame their options differently, the equations are combined differently, resulting in the different graphs.[3] To get a feel for this difference, the inner dialog that might accompany the top panel is: "Should I get high today?" The hypothetical user in the bottom panel might say, "Do I want to be high all the time, just on Saturday nights, or none of the time?" Figure 6.2, then, shows how the manner in which choices are framed affects the likelihood of drug use.

The top panel shows that local choice led to an all-out binge in which every choice was a drug choice. The value of the drug was always higher than the value of any nondrug activity so that it was always chosen. In contrast, the bottom panel shows that global choice led to abstinence—the drug was never chosen. Same preferences, same drugs, yet depending on how the options were framed, different choices. Indeed, not just different choices, but the opposite outcomes: an everyday drug binge or abstinence. To see how this is possible, we need to examine the graph in some detail.

First consider drug use from a day-to-day perspective (top panel). The horizontal axis is the number of days an individual chose to use a drug in the last thirty days. As in the restaurant graph, the horizontal axis represents a moving window. It shows the most recent thirty choices, not necessarily the first thirty opportunities to use the drug. The vertical axis lists the current values of drug days and nondrug days. These values changed as a function of how frequently the drug was used. The decrease in the value of the drug represents tolerance. The decrease in the value of the nondrug activities represents the drug-related problems that are referred to or alluded to in the *DSM*. Intoxication and withdrawal impede normal functioning, particularly the activities that comprise conventional social situations and work. Someone who is high on heroin or who is going through withdrawal symptoms cannot properly tend to family responsibilities or fulfill most work expectations. There are also indirect drug-related problems. These include legal consequences, such as an arrest record, and the stigma that often accompanies heavy drug use. Consequently, the value of the drug, although declining, remained higher than the value of the nondrug activities. In the end, this dynamic process stabilized at exclusive preference for the drug, even though the value of the drug had declined more than 60 percent.

The horizontal axis in the global-choice (bottom) panel is the same as in the local-choice panel: the number of drug days is the most recent thirty days. The vertical axis is the value of each possible thirty-day sequence of drug days and nondrug days. For example, for a horizontal axis value of 12, the vertical axis displays the value of 12 drug days and 18 nondrug days. (As in Figure 6.1, order is not represented.) The thirty-day sequence with the highest value was the one that contained no drug days. Thus, in the hypothetical situation represented by Figure 6.2, someone who framed his or her choices globally would never use drugs. Note that the difference is not because the global bookkeeper liked drugs any less than the local bookkeeper. Our hypothetical subject liked them just as much. Rather, when the choice was between different thirty-day samples, which can be interpreted as a choice among competing lifestyles, the one that did not contain drugs was considered best. This, in turn, was a function of the equations that generated the graph. They were selected to make the point that as a function of the frame of reference, voluntary behavior could lead to two utterly different patterns of drug use. For a nondrug example of the psychology represented by the graphs, imagine someone who wants to be physically fit but who doesn't like to exercise. Since the goal is to be fit, thirty days at the gym is better than twenty-nine days at the gym. However, if the decision to go to the gym is made each morning at 6:30 A.M., this same person prefers an extra hour of sleep. The dilemma is probably familiar to at least some readers, and it often sets in motion defensive stratagems, such as arranging to go to the gym with a friend or placing alarm clocks away from the bed to prevent carrying out the choice called for by local bookkeeping.

Figure 6.2 is the simplest possible graph of the relationships described in the *DSM* account of addiction. The values associated with actual drug use and nondrug activities would not change in a simple linear way, and the transition from low to moderate levels of drug use would probably involve an increase in the value of drug use and maybe even an increase in the value of some nondrug activities. Thus, a graph of actual drug use would be more complex than Figure 6.2. However, graphs that come at the end of this chapter and elsewhere (e.g., Heyman, 1996) reveal that more complex curves would not alter any of the conclusions that follow from Figure 6.2. When the choices include a commodity that has behavioral effects that are consistent with the *DSM* description of addiction, then the local equilibrium will be associated with markedly poorer outcomes relative to the global equilibrium.

Although highly simplified, Figure 6.2 captures key features of addiction. From the perspective of the bottom panel, the "person" represented in the top panel is self-destructive and excessive. This hypothetical subject always chose the drug, and this led to more than a 60 percent decrease in overall welfare (assuming no drug use at the start). But from the perspective of the top panel, every drug choice was the best choice. Figure 6.2, then, says that judgments regarding the nature of addiction, such as its self-destructive properties, are based on a global perspective. When drug users regret their past behavior (or anticipate future relapses), they too are taking a global perspective. When one of the options corresponds to the *DSM* account of an addictive drug, then choice can produce the worst possible outcome. This conclusion follows from nothing more than the three principles that characterize the responses to the restaurant problem and the *DSM* account of addiction.

This chapter began with the hypothesis that the principles that predict everyday choice also predict addiction. Figures 6.1 and 6.2 confirm the hypothesis. The pattern of choices in Figure 6.1 is consistent with the results of literally hundreds of studies (e.g., Davison & McCarthy, 1988; Williams, 1988), and the pattern of choices in Figure 6.2 is consistent with the *DSM* description of addiction. One way to put this is that addiction is the result of a mismatch between how choices are made and certain properties of addictive drugs (Herrnstein & Prelec, 1992). For example, in the local frame of reference the future and indirect consequences of current choices do not count. This "oversight" might not matter that much if the costs associated with a commodity are as apparent as its benefits. But for drugs, the costs are delayed, indirect, and uncertain. As a result, there is a misleading bias in the relationship between perceived costs and perceived benefits. The perceived costs are discounted, but the perceived benefits are not. Thus, the actual value of the drug is distorted in a way that promotes its further use. It is important to note that the distortion does not reflect pathology or some sort of cognitive deficit. Individuals typically make choices on the basis of the current values of the options. Moreover, it is quite likely that this is a reasonable approach under most circumstances. Some calculations suggest that under most circumstances the local equilibrium is not that different from the global equilibrium (e.g., Heyman, 1982, 1983), and the additional benefits provided by the global equilibrium may be somewhat smaller than indicated by the graphs in this book. This is because global bookkeeping is necessarily more complicated, and the costs associated with the complexity of the calculations were not included in the graphs (as it is not clear how to do so). Figures 6.1 and 6.2 then reveal that addiction is the result of the basic principles that apply to all voluntary action and the behavioral effects of addictive drugs. We need not assume disease or even abnormal decision making.

Why it is hard to quit. According to the bottom panel of Figure 6.2, a heavy user who switches to a global-choice perspective will stop using drugs. However, the graph also reveals that it would be difficult to maintain this new perspective. This is because the rewards associated with the global perspective accrue rather slowly, and at the beginning of abstinence the value of a nondrug day is less than the value of the most recent drug days (from a local perspective). These points deserve attention, as they help explain one of the apparent irrationalities of addiction. As drug use persists, it becomes harder and harder to understand because the value of the drug has declined and also the various costs have begun to take their toll. At the very least, drug use should decrease, but for addicts, it doesn't. Figure 6.2 helps makes this understandable. It shows that it is possible for the worst drug days to have a higher value than even an extended period of abstinence.

In the hypothetical situation in Figure 6.2, thirty or more days of drug use drives the value of the drug and the values of the competing activities to their lowest possible values. On this graph this is 120 units of pleasure for a thirty-day sequence or 4.0 units of pleasure a day. The units are arbitrary, but it helps to provide a numerical value to see what happens when drug use stops. Now assume that drug use comes to a halt for thirty days or more. The graphs show that abstinence affords 11.0 units of pleasure each day, a substantial improvement. However, it takes thirty days to reach this goal. Moreover, the graph also shows that it would take about thirteen days of not using drugs to experience a day that was as good as the worst drug day. This is because it takes about thirteen "moves" from the right end of the horizontal axis to push the value of abstinence above that of the worst drug day. Consequently, at a day-by-day level, abstinence starts off as worse than drug use. One implication of these calculations is that for someone who cannot forget how good drug use was, quitting requires a change in circumstances.

Figure 6.2 points to the hurdles that face someone who wants to quit, and it also suggests ways to quit. From a local bookkeeping perspective, quitting can only occur if there is a change in conditions that markedly reduces the value of the drug relative to the nondrug alternative. The biographical accounts presented in Chapter 3 are consistent with this prediction. Recall that in a number of the accounts, quitting was preceded by a change in economic conditions that markedly increased the drug's real price. Scott, Jessie, William Burroughs, and Patty could have kept using, but they would have had to spend their last dollars on heroin or cocaine to do so. They decided that it wasn't worth it. The other way to quit, according to Figure 6.2, involves experiences that promote a global bookkeeping perspective. The biographical accounts are also consistent with this perspective. When Patty pointed out that a steady diet of cocaine was at odds with her role as a mother and PTA member, she was shifting to a global frame of reference. This is because social roles identify a pattern of behavior, not a particular choice. You are not a "good" or "bad" mother on the basis of one day but on the basis of a consistent series of acts over many days. From this vantage point, cocaine was no longer a reasonable choice. Similarly, when Scott says that drug dealing was incompatible with his legitimate job, he was weighing two different sequences of choices or lifestyles. But the graph also shows that a shift in the frame of reference is not likely to be enough to quit. As described above, for situations similar to the one depicted by Figure 6.2, the first weeks of abstinence will not produce a day that has more value than the worst drug day. This means that quitting requires a steadfast commitment to the global approach to choice and a plan of action that erases reminders of the day-to-day pleasures of drug use. The graph also suggests that during the first weeks of abstinence, programs that made access to drugs impossible or greatly reduced their value, as methadone does for heroin, would be useful, particularly if they included measures that enhanced the value of nondrug alternatives.

Predicting Distinctive Features of Addiction

The vocabulary of relapse. Relapse and other forms of backsliding are often attended by a number of formulaic excuses. The following list will likely sound familiar: "It's a special occasion . . . It's just this one time . . . My friends are here for only one more weekend; when they go, I will stop drinking so much . . . It's the last time. Tomorrow, I'll turn over a new leaf . . . It's a once in a lifetime chance," and so on.

The common theme in these remarks is that the next occasion of drug use is unique and it is just for one more time. Interestingly, over a hundred years ago a similar list was compiled. William James, who is sometimes referred to as the first American experimental psychologist, documented the "drunkard's excuses" (1899). They echo the same themes as those listed above:

> He has made a resolve to reform, but he is now solicited again by the bottle . . . If he says that it is a case of not wasting good liquor already poured out, or a case of not being churlish and unsociable when in the midst of friends, or a case of learning something at last about a brand of whiskey which he never met before, or a case of celebrating a public holiday, or a case of stimulating himself to a more energetic resolve in favor of abstinence than any he has ever yet made, then he is lost. His choice of the wrong name seals his doom. But if, in spite of all the plausible good names with which his thirsty fancy so copiously furnishes him, he unwaveringly clings to the truer bad name, and apperceives the case as that of "being a drunkard, being a drunkard, being a drunkard," his feet are planted on the road to salvation. He saves himself by thinking rightly.

James's list shows that the "last time" and "special occasion" excuses were alive and well in the nineteenth century. This generality raises two questions. Why is relapse so often preceded by the statement that this is a "special occasion"? And why is a "special occasion" a good excuse to have another drink?

The excuse reflects an underlying dilemma. From a local perspective, the drug is the best choice; but from a global perspective, abstinence is the best choice. The ideal solution is to somehow do both. This is impossible, except in one situation. On the last choice in a series of choices, the distinction between the local and global perspectives disappears. The global perspective requires a continuing sequence of choices. When there is just one choice, only the local perspective applies. When a meteor is heading for Earth, it is okay to eat cheesecake.[4] Thus, if the situation can be framed as the "last time," then the dilemma dissolves. The same reasoning applies to "special occasions."

Of course, it is highly unlikely that the series of opportunities to use drugs again really came to a halt. Under these circumstances, the excuse will either be reiterated or the drug will simply be used with no excuses. In either case, the relapse is underway. Thus, the "last time" excuse establishes a frame of reference in which the drug is the right choice (assuming it really is the last time), but then when opportunities for drug use reoccur, the excuse implies that the local perspective is in charge—hence, a relapse.

Spontaneous recovery. Suppose that certain changes in circumstances, say the possibility of losing one's livelihood or the start of a new romantic relationship, influenced how drug users frame their options. If the frame of reference makes a big difference for choice, as in Figure 6.2, then a switch from a local to a global bookkeeping perspective will look like "spontaneous recovery." If it is also the case that choice plays a much more important role in addiction than in other psychiatric disorders, then spontaneous recovery will distinguish addiction from other disorders. The following observations support both suppositions.

First, the biographical accounts of drug use revealed that a number of the addicts quit all at once. Scott abruptly quit using heroin; Patty and Jessie abruptly quit using cocaine. Second, a computer search for the terms "spontaneous recovery" and "spontaneous remission" yielded about seven times as many hits for addiction and alcoholism than for obsessive compulsive disorder and Tourette's syndrome. Third, addiction is the only *DSM* psychiatric disorder that has been a source of new words for spontaneous recovery. The phrases "going cold turkey" and "kicking the habit" identify specific heroin withdrawal symptoms and were first used to refer to quitting heroin all at once. They are now used to describe quitting any drug—or habit—all at once, but these terms occur rarely if at all in association with other psychiatric disorders. It is not likely that anyone ever referred to recovery from obsessive compulsive disorder or schizophrenia as "going cold turkey." Thus, the idea that addiction involves voluntary drug use, and that voluntary behavior involves local- and global-choice equilibria, predicts the distinctive manner in which addiction sometimes ends as well as how people talk about addiction.

Voluntary addiction does not mean someone chooses to be an addict. The view that addicts are voluntary drug users is sometimes rejected on the grounds that "no one would choose to be an addict." The implication of this statement is that no one would choose the miseries usually associated with heavy drug use. However, Figure 6.2 does not say that someone chooses addiction. The top panel says that what the addict chooses is to use the drug one more time, nothing more. The point is that one day of heroin does not mean addiction, just as eating dessert once does not make one fat. Of course as the days accumulate, the characteristics of addiction emerge, and as the desserts accumulate, fat cells get bigger. From the local bookkeeping perspective, however, the options relate to the current situation, not a state of being. Consequently, a person who never chose to be an addict ends up an addict. Similarly, someone who has a second helping of dessert every night ends up twenty pounds heavier than he or she had planned. Thus, it is probably generally correct to say that no one would choose to be an addict, and this is what Figure 6.2 shows. The figure, though, adds the point that choices which create an undesirable way of life are made one day at a time; they are not made at the level of a lifestyle.

Explaining Consumerism and Excess

The analysis presented in this chapter applies to the tendency for people to do too much of anything that they like, not just drugs. This tendency is long and widely recognized. Aristotle preached "moderation in all things," something he would not have bothered with if excess were not a problem in Athens in the third century BC. Similarly, Henry David Thoreau would not have escaped to Walden Pond if nineteenth-century New England had not seemed too cluttered and materialistic. But despite this long history of criticism of excess, excess has persisted wherever there is wealth and may even be on the rise. According to recent reports,

Americans of all ages are getting fatter, houses are getting larger, and, before gas prices increased, cars were growing bigger and bigger. It seems fair to say that excessive consumption is an age-old problem and one that has increased over time.

In particular cases of excess, there are theories as to why it happens. The disease theory explains excessive drug use, and some have blamed advertising and marketing for overeating. However, history shows that concerns about excessiveness predate addictive drugs, advertising, and McDonald's. These observations suggest that a theory of excessive consumption should apply widely. It should explain too many shoes, too many sweaters, and the excesses of third-century Greece and nineteenth-century Concord, Massachusetts.

But there is no commonly accepted theory, and this is not by oversight. Both economics and behavioral biology imply that a theory of excess is not needed. According to economics, individuals and firms tend to end up at the global equilibrium. In cases where this is not achieved, the explanation is that some sort of mistake or bias is at play, not principle. According to biologists, organisms maximize fitness. This precludes persistently excessive consumption patterns. For both disciplines, excessive maladaptive consumption patterns are a kind of irrationality or accident; phenomena that do not fit the standard analyses.

In contrast, in the local/global analysis, excess is a fundamental feature of voluntary behavior. This was hinted at in the discussion of the restaurant problem, and it is a feature of Figures 6.1 and 6.2. In the restaurant problem, the local equilibrium was associated with too much Chinese food, and in the addiction graph, the local equilibrium was associated with too much drug. From a global bookkeeping perspective, the favorite item was consumed excessively. These are not special cases. Given a set of items, the local equilibrium implies that the one that is most favored is overconsumed. As shown next, this conclusion is a logical consequence of the relationship between the local equilibrium and the global equilibrium.

Recall that the global equilibrium identifies the ideal consumption level. Each item is consumed at just the right amount to insure that the overall benefits of consumption are maximized. Also notice that Figures 6.1 and 6.2 were drawn from the perspective of the good or activity that had the highest value prior to any consumption. For instance, the vertical axis in Figure 6.1 showed preferences for someone who liked Chinese food more than Italian food, and, accordingly, the horizontal axis was the number of Chinese meals. Similarly, Figure 6.2 showed someone who liked drugs more than the nondrug alternatives, and accordingly the horizontal axis depicted the number of drug choices. In both graphs, the local equilibrium is to the right of the global equilibrium. Since the global equilibrium defines the ideal consumption level, this means that the local equilibrium entails too much consumption of the favorite good—too much Chinese food and too many drugs. Figure 6.3 shows that these relations are quite general.

Figure 6.3 closely resembles the restaurant and heroin graphs. On the horizontal axis is the frequency of choices for the commodity that was initially liked best (prior to any choices). On the vertical axis are the choice-dependent changes in value. The curved lines show the choice-dependent changes in value for a commodity that replenishes and depletes according to exponential functions (Heyman, 1982, 2003). Despite the particular shape of the value curve and the distance between the local and global equilibrium, the local equilibrium is always to the right of the global equilibrium. This means that even when the local equilibrium is highly efficient (as measured by its close proximity to the global equilibrium), the favorite good is still consumed a little too much. Pirooz Vakili, a member of Boston University's College of Engineering, has derived a proof that confirms the implications of the graphs.[5]

Critics of consumerism have often blamed social institutions or "society." The analysis presented here does not deny that social forces play an important role in promoting excessive consumption levels. What it adds is the point that there would be excessive consumption even if advertising did not exist. As long as choices are made from the local perspective, and this is usually the perspective that people take, the favored good will be consumed excessively. Advertisers and merchants encourage this tendency, and conversely, ascetic movements counter this tendency.

Why Does Local Bookkeeping Persist?

Local choice has serious drawbacks. As just demonstrated, it sets the stage for addiction. The example was a drug. But for local choice, the problems posed by drugs apply to any substance or activity that undermines the competition and has immediate positive consequences accompanied by negative consequences that lag far behind. This category includes many foods, sex, gambling, and perhaps various computer games. These

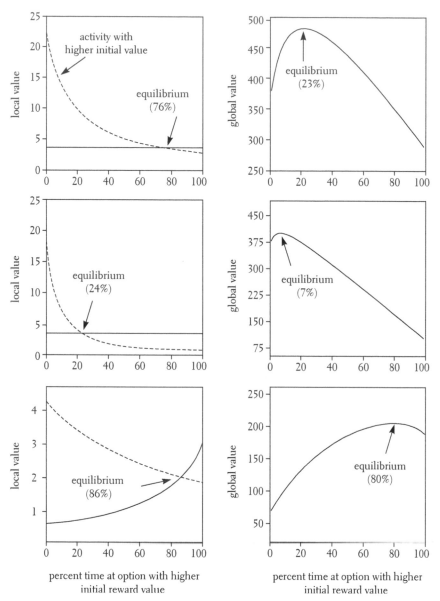

6.3 The relationship between the local and global equilibria for various commodities. The local equilibrium is always to the right of the global equilibrium. From the perspective of the global equilibrium, right panel, this means that local choice always involves consuming too much of the preferred item. Thus, the analysis of choice presented in this chapter says that individuals who stick to a local-choice strategy always overconsume their favorite item. The equations that generated the graph are similar to those I have used in earlier papers to model choice (e.g., Heyman & Luce, 1979; Heyman, 2003).

are well-known problems that many theories of choice address. There is also a subtle, possibly more costly drawback. In almost all ordinary situations, the local equilibrium provides a lower rate of overall benefits than does the global equilibrium.[6] Often the differences are quite small. But as we are almost always in a setting that offers more than one alternative, the differences should add up. Thus, everyday events as well as highly seductive opportunities lead local choice astray.

These observations say that the local perspective should give way to the global perspective. Learning is like natural selection. Thus, if local and global choice compete for the same niche, global choice should win. Nevertheless, in most studies the local equilibrium prevails (Davison & McCarthy, 1988; Williams, 1988). There are exceptions, however, and they provide insight into why the local equilibrium is dominant.

How to teach economic rationality. There are a handful of studies that explore the conditions that promote the global-choice equilibrium. The basic finding is that when the experimenter provided cues that were correlated with combinations of the competing outcomes—thereby suggesting the way options are organized in global bookkeeping—the subjects shifted toward the global equilibrium. Rachlin and his colleagues describe this as "patterning." In a study that illustrates this approach and the advantages of patterning, college students played a choice game that mimicked the properties of the addiction graph (Figure 6.2, Kudadjie-Gyamfi & Rachlin, 1996). There were two buttons. Pressing one earned more money on the current trial, but this reduced future rewards so that pressing the other button earned more money overall. Thus, one button was best from a local perspective (the current trial), but the other button was best from a global perspective (earnings over a series of ten trials). The basic finding was that choices varied as a function of how the trials were presented. When choice trials were separated by a fixed period of time (ten seconds), choices approximated the values predicted by the local equilibrium. When choice trials were presented in threes, separated by a long, fixed period of time (thirty seconds), choices shifted toward the global equilibrium. Three quick choices separated by a long interval established a rhythm or tempo that echoed the actual interdependence of the choices and outcomes. Thus, when the choice trials were presented as aggregates, the subjects made choices that reflected the more profitable aggregate structure of the options.

A somewhat similar study shows that it is even possible to teach pigeons to allocate responses in the manner predicted by the global equilibrium (Heyman & Tanz, 1995). Larry Tanz, then a graduate student in the Department of Psychology at Harvard, and I arranged for a light to go on when choice proportions approximated the global solution (so that it was correlated with higher reward rates). For instance, the combination of choices "8 left responses and 2 right responses" turned on the light. The pigeons, who had heretofore distributed their choices as called for by the local equilibrium, shifted to the more efficient global response pattern. That is, they learned to keep the light on. However, note that in this example, the environment provided the global solution. The pigeons did not have to calculate choice-dependent changes in reward value, they just had to keep the light on. The experimenters made the calculations and encouraged the pigeons to follow along by linking the light to a higher overall reward rate. The pigeons rapidly learned to re-allocate their choices so as to keep the light on (and earn more food).

Although it was possible to teach pigeons to allocate their responses as if they were choosing between "market baskets," thereby mimicking the hypothetical consumers in economic text books, humans are much better at finding the global equilibrium. In experiments with humans, some subjects typically discovered the global equilibrium without any overt instructions (e.g., Herrnstein et al., 1993). Also, recall that the restaurant problem tends to prompt a few global equilibrium solutions. To my knowledge, in experiments in which the local and global equilibria offer distinctly different outcomes, no other species has discovered the global equilibrium on their own (e.g., Herrnstein & Heyman, 1979; Heyman & Herrnstein, 1986). Pigeons and rats have to be explicitly taught, as in the pigeon study described above (also see Silberberg & Williams, 1974). The species differences are intriguing. They suggest that the capacity to reflect upon the options is one of the factors that distinguishes global choice from local choice.

Researchers have encouraged their subjects to take a global approach to choice by providing cues that correspond to the aggregate structure of the options in global choice. This is a way of saying that global choice is more cognitively demanding than local choice. It also points to a more subtle reason for why local choice is the more usual result.

The options in local choice are concrete and correspond to how things look. Local choice involves items that have clear physical outlines and activities that are easy to name. By definition, Italian and Chinese restaurants inhabit different localities and may even inhabit different neighborhoods. In contrast, the aggregates of global choice have no naturally occurring boundaries, but are abstractions. For example, there is no physical counterpart to the ideal combination of meals in the restaurant problem. Rather, the competing aggregated meal sequences are played out in the imagination. Put another way, local choice corresponds to the natural fracture lines of perception; global choice does not. Of course, it is possible to concoct new categories that correspond to global-choice aggregates. This is what we do when we create schedules, plans, diets, and so on. But this takes imagination and forethought. Thus, local choice persists despite its drawbacks because it is simpler and the options of local choice are consistent with how things look and their customary labels.

How Rational Is Voluntary Behavior?

According to economics, individuals and firms either maximize overall well-being or are on the road to doing so. This result is built into the economic model of choice. It is a global maximizing process. In biology it is often assumed that evolution guarantees optimal outcomes. In both disciplines voluntary behavior guarantees success. This chapter tells a different story. It shows that it is always possible for choice proportions to stabilize at a less-than-optimal equilibrium. When this occurs, the analysis of consumerism showed that the commodity that was initially the favorite was overconsumed. The degree of excess depends on the distance between the local equilibrium and the global equilibrium. It is my hunch that for most commodities this distance is rather small, so that the level of excess is small. It is, however, an ever-present inefficiency, and one that has been overlooked. The analysis also showed that ambivalence is logically inherent to voluntary behavior and will be an actual presence for individuals who are aware of the current values of the available items and are also aware of the influence that their choices are going to have on the future values of the items. This is disconcerting, particularly when the two approaches to choice call for conflicting courses of action—from one perspective, one is always doing the wrong thing. Finally, although global choice is the "natural approach" in economic texts, it is out of step with the world in the sense that the options, referred to in this chapter as "aggregates" and in economics textbooks as "bundles" or "market baskets," have no naturally occurring counterparts. For example, one widely used textbook describes hypothetical consumers as choosing between competing bundles of "pounds of cheese" and "boxes of rubber bands" (Baumol & Blinder, 1994). The description includes a graph that displays all possible aggregates of these two items: 3 pounds of cheese and 2 boxes of rubber bands versus 4.5 pounds of cheese and one box of rubber bands, and so on. But bundles of rubber bands and pounds of cheese do not seem a very likely category—"I will have 6 boxes of rubber bands with my cheese, please." The example suggests that the point is to introduce the student to an approach to studying choice, but not to describe what people actually do.

Research supports this darker image of voluntary behavior. In labs and in natural settings, choice proportions approximated the local, not the global equilibrium. This in turn suggests that addiction and other forms of excess should be quite common. However, societies cannot function well if their members are so easily seduced by "specious" rewards (Ainslie, 1975). These considerations suggest that there is a role for measures that protect people from themselves, one of the issues that will be explored in the next chapter.

The first five chapters presented research findings. In this chapter, the approach was different. The discussion was based on three self-evident principles that pertain to all voluntary activities and their logical implications. The logical implications predicted the pattern of choices found in experiments and addiction. The local equilibrium, equivalent to the matching law result, summarizes the results of hundreds of studies on choice; the global equilibrium is equivalent to the predictions of economic analyses. One of the new features of this analysis is the idea that voluntary behavior involves both the local and global equilibria. This means that the contingencies that govern voluntary action are inherently ambiguous, that choice can stabilize at suboptimal outcomes (from the perspective of the global equilibrium), and that choices are inherently labile, subject to change if the frame of reference changes. The restaurant example (Figure 6.1) suggests that local choice often produces reasonably good outcomes, but the drug example (Figure 6.2) shows that when one of the options undermines the value of competing options, local choice can drive overall welfare to its lowest possible level. Behaviorally toxic commodities are relatively recent phenomena. Opium smoking and potent distilled alcohol solutions did not become widely available until the sixteenth and seventeenth centuries. If addiction is inherent to voluntary behavior, then as soon as behavioral toxic substances appear, addiction should appear also. Historically, this is what happened.

The empirical research and the logic of voluntary behavior (the three principles and their implications) lead to the same conclusions. Both show addiction as choice, and choice as somewhat treacherous. The logic, though, has the advantage of generating new predictions. These include an explanation of the excuses that accompany relapse, the association between spontaneous recovery and addiction, and the age-old problems of consumerism and excessive consumption levels. According to the analysis presented in this chapter, these are related observations, each revealing the competing influences of local and global choice.

Although this chapter reveals that voluntary behavior involves pitfalls and that choosing what is best can actually lead to the worst overall possible outcome, the next chapter reveals that there is also a "bright" side to voluntary behavior. Figures 6.1 and 6.2 also suggest that simply engaging in voluntary action has the potential to encourage individuals to reformulate their options in more abstract terms and to exercise self-control. This discussion emerges in the process of addressing two long-standing issues in addiction: the properties that make a substance addictive and the individual differences that increase the likelihood of using addictive drugs in a self-destructive manner.

7

VOLUNTARY BEHAVIOR:
AN ENGINE FOR CHANGE

Chocolate is delicious and widely available, yet surveys suggest that only about one percent of the population eats chocolate every day (e.g., Rossner, 1997; Seligson et al., 1994). In contrast, about 50 percent of the enlisted men stationed in Vietnam during the war who tried an opiate just once went on to become heavy users. They reported cravings and withdrawal symptoms, and when it was time to leave Vietnam, many kept using despite penalties such as a forced stay in detox and a delayed departure for home (Robins et al., 1975; Robins, 1993). It is not likely that many chocolate lovers would put chocolate ahead of leaving war-torn Vietnam and returning to family and friends. Some might argue that opiate users in Vietnam were responding to extreme, even unique, circumstances. But in an inner-city St. Louis, Missouri, neighborhood, the addiction rate for young men who experimented with heroin just a few times was also greater than 50 percent (Robins & Murphy, 1967). Why is heroin so much more likely to lead to addiction than chocolate? Neuroscientists have an answer. According to research papers and reviews, what makes a drug addictive is dopamine. The current consensus is that addictive drugs share the common property of increasing the effectiveness of dopamine, a neurotransmitter that is associated with reward and movement. However, there are reasons to think that this account is at best incomplete.

Dopamine—a Biological Common Denominator?

A *Science News* article on addiction that appeared during the height of the most recent war on drugs (Hendricks, 1988) led with the line: "Just say dopamine." The article summarized the results from a series of studies in which rats self-administered or were injected with nicotine, alcohol, stimulants, or opiates. These drugs bind to different receptors, so they have different pharmacological effects and different psychological effects. Yet they are all addictive, and, as the article emphasized, they all increased brain levels of dopamine.

Reflecting on the rat studies, Roy Wise, a neuroscientist who did pioneering work on the role of dopamine in behavior, commented, "These results confirm [my] theory that dopamine is the common denominator of drug addiction." In support of Wise's comments, the 1988 rat results have been replicated many times, and the more recent studies include humans as well as rodents in their subject pool. An article published in 2004 in NIDA's monthly account of important research findings summarizes the dopamine research as follows (NIDA Notes, vol. 19, April): "In the past few decades, scientists have firmly established that the desire to take drugs has a biological basis in fluctuation in levels of the brain chemical dopamine." Scores if not hundreds of other publications have made this same point.

To be sure, many addictive drugs lead to changes in dopamine levels. The experimental findings are not in dispute. Rather, the problem with the dopamine theory is that dopamine does not distinguish addictive substances from rewarding but nonaddictive substances. Many if not all events that can function as rewards for voluntary behavior elicit the release of dopamine in the nucleus accumbens. The list includes consummatory activities, such as eating; nonconsummatory rewards, such as stimulating exercises; and even pleasurable cognitive activities, such as looking at cartoons (Heyman & Seiden, 1985; Mobbs et al., 2003; Stellar et al., 1983). Looking at cartoons is rewarding, but it is safe to say it has rarely if ever become an addiction. Moreover, even aversive events increase dopamine levels. In rats, a tail pinch elicits avoidance and the release of dopamine in the nucleus accumbens (e.g., D'Angio et al., 1987), but no rat has become addicted to getting his or her tail pinched. There is not a specific relationship between dopamine and addictive drugs, and there is not even a specific relationship between dopamine and positive outcomes. John Salamone (1994), a neuroscientist who specializes in the biology of reward, concluded: "There is no evidence that the involvement of DA [dopamine] systems in emotion is selective for 'hedonia', 'euphoria' or other such emotions with positive valence" (p. 125). If dopamine does not have a selective relationship with positive rewards, then logic demands that it is not the factor that distinguishes addictive from nonaddictive rewards. At the very least there has to be more to the biology of addiction than dopamine.

Is There a Behavioral Common Denominator in Addiction?

On logical grounds there is no need to assume that addictive substances share some common biological and behavioral set of traits. Each addictive substance could lead to an addictive pattern of behavior in its own way. For instance, the same computer algorithm can run on various hardware, whether electronic relays, cathode ray tubes, or silicon transistors. Nevertheless, there is some reason to think that there may be a rather small number of common behavioral and biological features that together distinguish addictive substances from other rewarding substances. This hypothesis follows from two observations. First, there is an immense number of highly rewarding and compelling activities and substances that are relatively easy to obtain. In addition to obvious rewarding substances and activities, such as foods, sports, sex, the arts, and home projects, the Internet lists thousands of topics and activities that attract tens of thousands of enthusiasts, from model trains to Civil War battles, to movie posters, to the Dead Sea Scrolls. Second, despite the immense number of rewarding substances and activities, the *DSM* lists only twenty or so addictive substances and one addictive activity (gambling). Since the list is so short relative to how long it would be if even a fraction of the many substances and activities people enjoy were addictive, the list of properties that make addiction possible must also be short. In Chapter 6, Figure 6.1 showed rewarding but nonaddictive substances, and Figure 6.2 showed a rewarding and addictive substance. Thus, we can use Figure 6.2, the addiction graph, to identify the factors that distinguish addictive substances.

According to Figure 6.2, an addictive substance has immediate benefits and hidden costs. It undermines the value of competing substances and activities. There are also two properties that are consistent with Figure 6.2 but were not discussed in Chapter 6. Substances that undermine global bookkeeping have greater addiction potential, and substances that are relatively immune to consumption-dependent decreases in value will also have greater addiction potential. An important corollary of this list is that if it captures "addictiveness," then most highly rewarding but nonaddictive substances and activities will not have these properties. They may, in fact, have just the opposite capacities. For example, highly rewarding but nonaddictive goods may increase the value of competing substances and activities, thereby setting in motion competing inhibitory forces. The following discussion tests these ideas. The goal is to see if the model of addiction presented in the last chapter, Figure 6.2, provides insight into the properties that distinguish addictive and nonaddictive rewards.

Behavioral toxicity. A substance is behaviorally toxic when it poisons the field, making everything else relatively worse. Conventional goods and activities are not behaviorally toxic; they are neutral or enhance the value of other activities and goods. For instance, as an individual fulfills his or her primary economic and physical needs, the current values of leisure activities increase and become more accessible (e.g., affordable). Conversely, as more time is spent in conventional leisure activities, the current value of day-to-day responsibilities increases, either because they need to be attended to or because they have become interesting again. There are also more subtle interactions, particularly for professions that go to some length to honor success. For instance, as an academic's publications increase, the number of invitations to serve on committees, give talks, review papers, and participate in various other professional activities increases. The common denominator of these added-on, "honorary" duties is that they reduce the time that can be spent in the activity that brought success. In sum, conventional goods and activities increase the value of competing goods and activities, and this establishes a negative feedback loop that decreases the frequency of conventional activities, particularly the more successful ones.

As described in the *DSM* and Chapter 6, the relationship between the illicit addictive drugs and competing activities is just the opposite. Intoxication and withdrawal interfere with the current value of everything but drug use. Also, in contrast to nonaddictive but rewarding activities, there is no way to be successful. No one is asked to be on a committee because he or she is good at smoking cigarettes or shooting heroin. Thus, rewarding but nonaddictive substances promote competing activities, whereas addictive substances undercut competing activities.

Temporal and probabilistic disparities in costs and benefits. Goods and activities differ in terms of the timing and certainty of their costs and benefits. For medicines, particularly bad-tasting ones, the costs are certain and come right away, whereas their benefits are uncertain and delayed. Consequently, they are underconsumed. For addictive substances, the temporal patterns and certainty of costs and benefits is just the opposite. Their benefits are certain and virtually instantaneous, whereas their costs are uncertain, and when they do occur, they are delayed. There is an excellent chance (about nine in ten) that a heavy drinker will not get cirrhosis of the liver, and if an alcoholic's liver does go bad it usually takes at least ten years from the start of heavy drinking (e.g., Lelbach, 1975). For cigarette smokers, the chance of contracting a serious smoking-related disease is less than certain, and for someone who started smoking in his or her early teens the disease will not show up until well into middle age. Because of these dynamics, the current value of a medical treatment, particularly an unpleasant one, underestimates its true value, whereas the current value of an addictive drug greatly overestimates its true value. Thus, medicines are underconsumed and addictive drugs are overconsumed.

George Ainslie (1975) labeled substances and activities with delayed or otherwise hidden costs "specious" rewards. This is an apt label. From the perspective of current choice, specious rewards have high value (because of immediate benefits and hidden costs), whereas from the perspective of global choice, their effective value is their true value because the costs have as much weight as the benefits.

Natural, self-inhibiting feedback loops. Conventional activities are usually directly self-inhibiting. Physical activities lead to fatigue, mental activities lead to boredom, food is satiating, and sex is associated with refractory periods. These properties are immediate and thus decrease the reward's current value. In contrast, addictive drugs do not cause fatigue or satiation. Tolerance, of course, reduces their value, but tolerance is not nearly as immediate as satiation or fatigue, and for heroin and alcohol, tolerance is offset by withdrawal symptoms. Thus, nonaddictive rewards tend to trigger processes that reduce their own current value to a greater extent than do addictive substances, tolerance notwithstanding.

Global choice and intoxication. The properties listed up to this point make a difference from the perspective of local choice, which is to say, from the perspective of the substance or activity's current value. In contrast, from the perspective of global choice, hidden and delayed costs are visible. Indeed, from the perspective of global choice they are not seductive sirens but warning bells. Thus, global choice serves a prophylactic function, guarding against excess. However, global bookkeeping can be derailed. As described in the previous chapter, it is a reasoning process that involves complex estimates of the costs and benefits of present and future consequences. Intoxicating substances undermine reason. In particular, intoxication reduces the ability to perceive far-off potential consequences and thereby enhances the value of the most immediate and salient stimuli (e.g., Steele & Josephs, 1990). According to the account of voluntary action developed in this and the last chapter, then, intoxicating substances are likely to be addictive. In support of this inference, there are no intoxicating substances that are not considered addictive, and all but one addictive substance is intoxicating (tobacco is the exception). Thus, intoxication distinguishes almost all addictive and nonaddictive substances, and the reason for this demarcation is that intoxication nullifies one of the major deterrents to addiction—global choice.

There is no shortage of highly rewarding substances and activities. However, fewer than two dozen appear in the *DSM* as addictive. Those that are addictive differ in distinctive ways from those that are not. They display one or more of the following properties: they are behaviorally toxic, they are specious, they are not strongly self-inhibiting, and they are intoxicating.

The Special Case of Cigarettes

To varying degrees these four traits characterize addictive substances and distinguish them from those that are rewarding but not addictive. Opiates, stimulants, and alcohol are intoxicating, behaviorally toxic, virtually instantaneously rewarding, and specious in that their costs are delayed and uncertain. But what about cigarettes? They are considered highly addictive, yet they are missing two of the characteristics that distinguish addictive substances from rewarding, nonaddictive ones. They are not intoxicating, and prior to the anticigarette legislation, which started in the late 1960s, they were not behaviorally toxic—smoking did not undermine competing nondrug activities. As exceptions promise to provide insight into the condition under which a general rule holds, cigarettes deserve our attention, although this book is largely concerned with illegal drugs.

One way to explain why cigarettes fail to fit the model is to say that cigarettes are not really addictive. In support of this approach, the authors of the landmark 1964 U.S. Surgeon General's Report on the health risks of smoking stated that smoking was not an addiction but a "habit" (p. 354). They explained the distinction in terms of withdrawal symptoms. Their point was that cigarette withdrawal did not measure up—an irritation, perhaps, but nothing like the distress that accompanies heroin and alcohol withdrawal (U.S. Surgeon General's Advisory Committee on Smoking and Health, 1964). Today's experts do not agree with the 1964 consensus on the addictive nature of cigarettes, but this is beside the point. Heavy, habitual smoking is a self-destructive form of voluntary behavior and thus the local/global analysis of choice should explain it. Indeed, to simplify the presentation, let us assume that cigarette smoking is properly called an "addiction," and that cigarettes are not behaviorally toxic, as was true until the recent prohibitions were put into effect. The challenge, then, is to explain why smoking is addictive when it is neither intoxicating nor behaviorally toxic.

Behaviorally toxic substances and activities maintain their edge over competing alternatives by undermining them. Given a local frame of reference for making choices, this leads to high levels of overconsumption (e.g., Figure 6.2). How, then, do cigarettes maintain an advantage over competing activities when they are not behaviorally toxic? Cigarettes lose their reward value over the course of the day so that the frequency of smoking should decline after the first few morning cigarettes. Yet many smokers stick to a steady rate of one to two cigarettes an hour from morning to night. This turns out to make sense if we revisit the nature of reward and choice.

Choice depends on context. The relative value of the competing options depends both on their intrinsic properties as well as the properties of the competition. If the context has little to offer, even unsubstantial activities and substances become the best choice. For example, in prisons and similar institutions, trivial objects become the source of life-and-death fights. Thus, the likelihood of choosing to engage in an activity increases as its context declines in value. With this is mind, consider the context in which smoking takes place.

As the ads pointed out (and was the case), smoking goes along with virtually all imaginable activities. Magazines and movies depicted smokers at their office desks, on horseback, in bed, riding in cars, riding on motorcycles, and even in scuba-diving gear, hanging off the side of a boat (with mask off). That smoking could accompany so many activities suggests that it didn't get in the way. And if it didn't get in the way of such a varied array of activities, then it had no competition. Smoking filled a niche that was home to few if any other activities. Or, and this is probably more accurate, smoking filled a niche that it created. For instance, prior to smoking there was no activity that accompanied horseback riding, driving, working at the office, and socializing. Thus, smoking occupied a niche which it had all to itself. This meant that even if smoking was not particularly rewarding, it would nevertheless remain the first choice from a local perspective. Since there are no competitors to undermine it, smoking doesn't need to be behaviorally toxic to maintain its edge.

Smoking's other addictive properties are like those of other drugs. It provides immediate pleasures and uncertain and greatly delayed costs. Indeed, given that smoking-related illnesses take years to develop and do so with some uncertainty, smoking is probably the most specious of all addictive substances. This analysis also makes predictions about the persistence of smoking. If smoking became so widespread because it filled a niche that had no competitors, then the introduction of just one inhibiting factor should lead to a marked decrease in its frequency. That is, the increase from zero to one inhibiting factor should make more of a difference than the increase from n to n plus one inhibiting factors. The recorded history of smoking prevalence in the United States beginning in 1910 shows the predicted pattern. In 1964, when the Surgeon General's Report linked smoking to cancer, the trend toward smoking abruptly reversed and has been steadily decreasing ever since. Tens of millions of smokers have quit, and the overall prevalence is less than half of what it was in 1964 (e.g., Heyman, 2003; USDHHS, 1990, 1994). But smoking is still legal, and the decline in smoking began virtually with the publication date, prior to the warning labels, prohibitions on where smoking can occur, and high taxes. What was new was the official consensus regarding the health risks of smoking. The experts agreed that smoking caused cancer. The implication was that if you continued to smoke, you were behaving irresponsibly. For large numbers of people, this message was enough motivation to quit.

Why Are All Addictive Substances Drugs?

There is nothing in the local/global account of addiction that says the focus of an addiction has to be a drug. Yet when it comes to addictive substances, the APA diagnostic manual lists only drugs. This, some critics say, ignores nondrug "addictions," such as such as overeating, overshopping, and so on. However, I think that there is a good reason why the *DSM* lists only drugs (with the exception of gambling). Drugs, as demonstrated below, are better than any other substances or activities at producing the effects that the local/global analysis of choice says are addictive. Drugs are more likely than any other substance or activity to produce behaviorally toxic effects, to function as specious rewards, to not inhibit their own consumption, and to derail global cost-benefit analysis. The brief overview of how drugs work, presented at the end of Chapter 2, shows why this is the case.

Recall that psychoactive drugs alter the functioning of neurons, which in turn alters consciousness, action, and affect. Drugs produce these effects because the mode of interneuronal communication is biochemical, and drugs are biochemicals.[1] It is possible to take drugs in amounts that dwarf those of their naturally occurring counterparts. This is what makes psychoactive drugs so attractive and so dangerous. It is easy to take heroin and other psychoactive agents in doses that produce hedonic effects that cannot be duplicated by nondrug experiences. For instance, recall that one of the themes in Chapter 3 was that heroin users felt that they could not put their drug reactions into words. From the perspective of local choice, uniqueness provides an advantage. But the drug doses that produce these unique psychological states are toxic and destabilizing. They trigger processes that restore the predrug equilibrium. This results in tolerance and withdrawal. The positive hedonic effects occur virtually instantaneously because the drug is acting directly on the nervous system, whereas the negative effects occur much later because they depend on reactions to the initial drug effects and are cumulative in nature. In addition, receptor binding does not trigger satiation for the drug—although it might do so for commodities that compete with the drug, as is the case for stimulant-induced anorexia. In short, drugs are more likely than other substances to display the traits that are so seductive from a local-choice perspective. They are the most specious of all substances, the most behaviorally toxic of all substances, the least self-satiating, and the most likely to derail global-choice cost-benefit analyses. Hence, drugs are the most likely substances to become the focus of an addiction.

Do addictive drugs produce cognitive deficits? Illicit drug users often score lower on cognitive tests than do subjects who have not been heavy drug users (Jovanovski et al., 2005; Mintzer & Stitzer, 2002; Solowij et al., 2002). Some have interpreted this result as demonstrating drug-induced cognitive deficits (e.g., Bolla et al., 1998; Lundqvist, 2005). This could explain why it is difficult to quit using drugs; or if there were individual differences in the susceptibility to these cognitive deficits, why there were individual differences in quitting. However, some researchers have found little or no evidence that addictive drugs produce persistent cognitive failings (e.g., Rapeli et al., 2005; Selby & Azrin, 1998). The disparate results reflect the difficulties in determining whether the cognitive differences are a function of drug use or the correlates of drug use. As noted earlier, drug users, particularly those who are most likely to participate in research studies, often suffer from psychiatric disorders that could themselves have cognitive correlates, and, of course, the cognitive differences could easily have been in place before heavy drug use began. One way to resolve the problem of determining whether a particular outcome reflects drug use or the correlates of drug use is to study the outcome in twins who have different drug-use histories. If both twins show the outcome, then it must be independent of drug use itself. If, though, the outcome shows up in just the drug-using twin, then it is a direct pharmacological effect or in some way related to the onset of drug use. Two studies conducted at Harvard Medical School used the twin methodology to evaluate the effects of illicit drugs on cognition (Lyons et al., 2004; Toomey et al., 2003). In each study one twin had a history of drug abuse and the other did not. To insure that differences did not reflect withdrawal symptoms, the criteria were for lifetime rather than current use. The primary drugs were marijuana (Lyons et al., 2004) and cocaine or amphetamine (Toomey et al., 2003). Each group participated in more than fifty different cognitive tests.

The basic finding was that the twins performed similarly on almost all the tests. In the study that examined the cognitive effects of marijuana use, the twins performed differently on three of fifty-six texts, and in the study that examined the effects of stimulants on cognition, they scored differently on nine of fifty-six tests. In six, the twin without a history of drug abuse had the significantly higher score; in three, the twin with a history of drug abuse scored higher. In both studies there was no correlation between level of performance and amount of drug use. The primary sign of pharmacological action—a dose response effect—was missing. Thus, the two studies that employed the best control conditions are among those that failed to find significant drug-related differences in cognition.

However, the Harvard Medical School twin research should not be taken as the final word. The subjects were rather high functioning, having completed on average two years of college, and had not abused drugs for a year or more prior to their participation in the project. Perhaps there were residual but temporary deficits, and perhaps a less-educated, lower-functioning population would show drug-induced cognitive deficits. For now, however, the hypothesis that certain drugs are addictive because they produce cognitive deficits that interfere with decision making remains an intriguing, but not established, possibility. Thus, the previous summary stands. The distinguishing properties of addictive substances are that they undermine competing rewards, they provide immediate pleasure but delayed, hard-to-detect costs, they are not directly satiating, and they are intoxicating. Not all addictive drugs express each of these properties to the same extent, but stimulants, opiates, and alcohol produce these effects to a greater extent than do other substances and activities. Cigarettes are not intoxicating or particularly rewarding, relative to other addictive drugs, but make up for these "deficiencies" by filling a niche that until recently had no competition.

It seems highly improbable that there is just one biological factor that accompanies this suite of traits. Indeed, there may be a number of biological pathways for each of the four traits. It is virtually certain that alcohol and opiates alter consciousness in different ways, and current research does not rule out multiple biological pathways to pleasure, the current focus on dopamine notwithstanding. Thus, the properties that distinguish addictive substances from rewarding but nonaddictive ones may prove simpler to describe at the behavioral level than at the biological level.

Why Aren't There More Addicts?

According to recent nationwide surveys, about 95 percent of Americans who used an addictive drug one or more times did not become addicted to it, and for alcohol the percentage who drank but did not become alcoholic was about 85 percent (Conway et al., 2006; Hasin et al., 2007; SAMHSA, 2003; Stinson et al., 2005). In Chapter 2, I remarked that these numbers were surprising; they still are. Pharmacological research offers no reason for drug use not to proceed to drug abuse. Similarly, the local versus global analysis of choice implies that drug use should usually lead to addiction. Both pharmacological and choice-based accounts of addiction agree: there should be a lot more addicts than the surveys report. Possibly scientific epidemiology is not up to the task of accurately reporting addiction. However, even if the actual numbers were several times greater than the official estimates, they would still fall short of expectations. There should be a lot more addicts.

The next section of this chapter explores why so many people are able to resist addictive drugs. The goal is to identify individual differences that affect whether drug use graduates to drug abuse. The local versus global analysis of choice will guide the search. According to the analysis of choice, there should be two types of individual differences, those that influence local choice and those that influence the likelihood of taking a global-choice perspective. Those that influence local choice should tend to make drugs less rewarding. This is because from a local perspective the drug is likely to have more value than its alternatives. An example of local deterrence was given in Chapter 2 in the discussion of the emergence of opiate addiction in China. Recall that many Asians avoid alcohol. They inherit a gene that produces a toxic reaction to alcohol. Those with this allele rarely binge drink or become alcoholics (e.g., Luczak et al., 2001). According to the analysis presented in the previous chapter, the gene reduces the immediate value of alcohol so that it is rarely preferred. The next section of this chapter explores whether there are analogous processes in place that inhibit illicit drug use. For example, there might be genes that make cocaine less rewarding. Individual differences that function at the level of global choice include processes that affect decision making directly. This is because the global-choice perspective implies abstinence or controlled drug use, hence any process that promotes global choice will automatically reduce the likelihood of addiction. For example, genetic differences that promote more abstract decision making should promote global bookkeeping, which in turn implies controlled drug use. Thus, the research literature should show a negative correlation between measures of cognition and the likelihood that drug use leads to addiction.

Local-Choice Individual Differences
There is evidence of genetic individual differences in illicit drug use (e.g., Tsuang et al., 2001). In contrast to the literature on alcohol, though,

little is known regarding the steps from DNA to heroin and cocaine use. Genetic differences could influence opiate metabolism, turning heroin into a toxin, or they could affect decision making such that future consequences were given more weight. Less obvious but perhaps more important are individual variations that produce differences in social relations, which in turn affect the immediate value of addictive drugs. There are three steps to this line of reasoning. Social relations, such as the likelihood of divorce, reflect differences in temperament and personality; differences in temperament and personality bear the stamp of both experience and heredity (Eysenck, 1980; Keller et al., 2005; Newcomb, 1986); and social relations operate at the local level. Taken together, these observations suggest that a robust measure of individual differences in social relations will predict individual differences in drug use.

Marriage: The antidrug relationship. Frequent illicit drug use is incompatible with most occupations, with family responsibilities, and with ties to friends who are pursuing licit goals. Of these relations, the individual the drug user puts most at risk is his or her spouse and other "significant others." Members of a household depend on one another, but it is not possible to depend on someone who puts drugs in front of domestic responsibilities. The threat posed by a partner who uses drugs heavily is great and immediate and is often responded to in kind with threats, arguments, tirades, pleading, and various forms of abuse. Of course not all significant others will react negatively to addiction and its warning signs. There may be unique arrangements that accommodate drug use in a partner, but spouses and potential spouses are the individuals most likely to react negatively to drug use, and they are also the ones most likely to do so in a visceral, immediate, and punitive manner.[2] Figure 7.1 tests these ideas. It shows the relationship between marriage and various psychiatric disorders, including drug abuse and drug addiction, among the 20,000 or so informants that participated in the Epidemiologic Catchment Area survey (Robins & Regier, 1991). The subjects, as described in Chapter 2, were selected so as to reflect the demographic characteristics of the United States for individuals 18 years old and older.

Marital status for a number of representative psychiatric disorders, including abuse and dependence, appears on the horizontal axis. On the vertical axis is the percentage of married and single individuals for each diagnosis. The prediction is that the percentage of those married will be

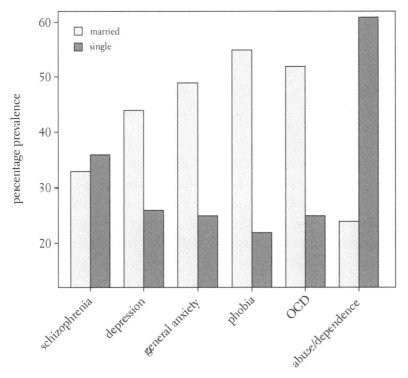

7.1 Prevalence of active cases of different psychiatric disorders as a function of marital status. Data are from the ECA study; Table 13.14 in Robins & Regier, 1991.

lowest for drug disorders. The results agree. Approximately 60 percent of those who were currently drug dependent or drug abusers were single, whereas about 25 percent were married. The rest were divorced or living with a partner with whom they did not have a legal bond ("cohabitation"). The percentages for the nondrug disorders were usually just the reverse. More than 50 percent of those with OCD were married, whereas 24 percent were single. One possible explanation for this pattern is that the age of onset was much lower for the drug-use disorders. However, the age of onset results fail to explain the data. The median age of onset for drug abuse and dependence was 18, and for the other disorders, it varied from 10 to 25 years old. For instance, the median onset age for OCD was 20, and for schizophrenia it was 19. Thus, serious psychiatric symptoms and marriage were not incompatible, except for schizophrenia and drug disorders. The simplest interpretation is that heavy users of illicit drugs do not readily form enduring relationships. The likelihood of forming a relationship reflects more fundamental individual differences in temperament and personality. Thus, individual differences that affect social relations end up playing a role in illicit drug use. The sequence of events parallels the sequence of events linking alcohol metabolism and alcohol use. In both cases individual differences influence the immediate, tangible consequences of drug use, and these in turn influence the rate at which the drugs are used.

Global-Choice Individual Differences

Since the global equilibrium is the optimal distribution of choices, processes that promote global choice will promote either abstinence or controlled illicit drug use. As described next, some of these processes emerge as a function of voluntary behavior itself. That is, engaging in voluntary behavior promotes global choice.

Background 1: Ambivalence or change? One of the lessons of the analysis of responses to the restaurant problem is that the goals that guide choice can be ambiguous. There were occasions when from a different perspective, the Chinese and Italian restaurants were both the "best" choice. In Figure 6.2, the drug is always the best choice from a local perspective, but never the best choice from a global perspective. Ambiguity promotes ambivalence, regret, and even dread—we may realize that we are going to make the wrong choice. There is, however, another way to look at the ambiguities that attend voluntary action. If choice typically gravitates to the local equilibrium, then the global equilibrium is an ever-present opportunity and stimulus to improve one's welfare. This means that simply engaging in voluntary behavior provides opportunities to improve one's lot. Moreover, the manner in which this comes about can involve both cognitive and motivational processes so that engaging in voluntary behavior not only offers opportunities to improve one's lot, but also the opportunity for cognitive and motivational change. If this argument is correct, then cognition, self-control, and voluntary behavior are closely linked in ways that heretofore have not been discussed.

Background 2: The advantages of abstract options and self-control. Local choice is the default state. The local options are simpler, and as noted in the previous chapter, the local options correspond to perceptual experience, whereas global options have no naturally occurring forms. In practice, we invent schedules, plans, diets, and other abstractions to represent global options. For example, a schedule arranges a combination of events into various orders and planning involves comparing and choosing among the different schedules. This process is equivalent to what economists say consumers are doing when they choose among different market baskets, made up of different combinations of groceries, clothing, housing, and entertainment. In effect, schedules and diets are versions of the global graphs shown in the previous chapter. Like the graphs, they are abstract, and in the sense of being dependent on human effort, they are artificial. Thus, global choice involves a good deal of effort, bother, and artificiality.

There is, however, a payoff. Since the global equilibrium provides higher rates of reward, the processes that produce the global equilibrium earn higher rates of reward and are thereby strengthened. In the restaurant problem, reformulating the options into more abstract categories— meal plans instead of meals—earned dividends. There were also dividends for avoiding the currently higher-valued Chinese meal when this brought choice proportions closer to the choice proportion that maximized overall dining pleasure. Thus, there was an incentive for self-control as well as an incentive for reformulating the options in more abstract terms. Note that these incentives emerged as a function of the act of engaging in voluntary behavior; they were not tacked on by an external agent. Voluntary behavior offers the opportunity to improve one's situation absent any other changes in the situation. In the restaurant problem, it was possible to obtain more pleasure in eating out by rearranging the options; no change in the restaurants themselves was necessary. This in turn should strengthen the processes that lead to reformulating the options and carrying out the new strategy. Put another way, voluntary activities are not just means to their various ends but are in themselves engines for cognitive and motivational change.

These observations call for three distinctions. First, they show that for someone who does not start off at the global equilibrium, engaging in voluntary behavior is a learning opportunity. Whether or not learning takes place depends on the magnitude of the global advantage and other factors, but regardless of the details, it is the case that for anyone not at the global equilibrium, engaging in voluntary behavior is a chance to acquire new, more efficient patterns of responding. Second, given the role of cognitive capacities and patience in global choice, these capacities provide protection against addiction. Third, there is also the possibility that the advantages of abstract thought and self-control play a role in genetic change across generations. As most of what mammals do is voluntary, even small differences in cognition and patience have the opportunity to produce dividends that over time are quite sizeable. Thus, the incentives inherent in voluntary action might differentially favor phenotypes that are more apt at reframing options globally and more apt at acquiring techniques for avoiding choices based on current value. For instance, experiments show that children differ in their ability to avoid looking at a tempting treat if doing so brings about an even better treat (e.g., Mischel et al., 1992). These, admittedly, are speculations. Whether or not voluntary action actually functions as a process that pushes individuals toward more abstract thought and greater patience has not been evaluated. However, we can test the prediction that differences in impulsivity and cognition are correlated with differences in addiction rates.

Drug use and impulsivity. The Oxford English Dictionary defines "impulsivity" as acting "without reflection or forethought." As global choice requires both reflection and forethought, impulsivity should be positively correlated with drug use. Recent research supports this conclusion. In drug studies, a procedure known as "delay discounting" has become the standard approach for measuring impulsivity (e.g., de Wit & Richards, 2004). The experimenter arranges a situation in which the subjects choose between a sooner, smaller reward and a later, larger reward. Most people are biased in favor of the sooner reward even though it is smaller. There are, however, individual differences, and these differences correspond with drug use. Heavy smokers, heavy drinkers, and heroin addicts depreciated the larger, later rewards at higher rates than did the control subjects (Bickel et al., 1999; Kirby et al., 1999; Mitchell, 1999; Vuchinich & Simpson, 1998). For example, ten dollars a week from now was worth less for heroin addicts than for control subjects not using drugs. A study by Samantha Gibb and myself (Heyman & Gibb, 2006) suggests that, in part, these differences were in place prior to drug use.

The subjects were Harvard undergraduates who were moderate smokers (12 cigarettes per day), weekend smokers ("cigarette chippers"), or nonsmokers. The subjects are of interest because they had been smoking for only a few years, and by the pack-a-day standard, they were not heavy smokers. As it is unlikely that smoking causes impulsivity, group differences in impulsivity would most likely reflect predrug differences. The basic finding was that smokers discounted future amounts of money, e.g., twenty-nine dollars delivered thirty days from the experimental session, at higher rates than did nonsmokers and chippers. For instance, the smokers were more likely to choose nine dollars on the day of the experiment than wait thirty days for twenty-nine dollars. The study was not longitudinal, so it is not possible to definitively rule out smoking-induced changes in impulsivity, but several observations suggest that this view is not particularly plausible. First, as mentioned, the students were not heavy or long-term smokers. Second, there is little or no experimental evidence that smoking affects impulsivity. Third, everyday experience also suggests that smoking does not cause impulsivity. When people quit smoking, they do not report that they have become more patient, nor is this a common observation. Thus, the general finding that drug users scored higher on laboratory tests of impulsivity reflects in part at least predrug individual differences. This, in turn, is consistent with the prediction that individual differences in capacities that promote global choice will be correlated with individual differences in addiction.

Drug use, global choice, and cognition. In the previous chapter, it was pointed out that although choice typically conforms to the local equilibrium predictions, in experiments with humans, some individuals spontaneously discovered the choice proportion that earned the highest rate of reward (the global equilibrium). This capacity might reflect differences in cognition, and it might also identify individuals who do not become addicted. Brian Dunn and I tested these hypotheses in a study that recruited subjects from Boston-area drug clinics who had a history of long-term opiate and stimulant use (Heyman & Dunn, 2002). The control subjects were from the same neighborhoods as the drug users. They typically had used illicit drugs and alcohol but had not become heavy drug users. Thus, the groups differed in their susceptibility to heavy drug use.

The procedure provided monetary rewards. As in the experiment on patterning of choices (described in the previous chapter; Kudadjie-Gyamfi & Rachlin, 1996), the contingencies mimicked the addiction graph (Figure 6.2). There were two buttons. One earned more money on the current trial but less overall; the other earned more money over a series of three consecutive trials but less on each current trial. Thus, the button that earned less money on the current trial earned more money overall. As predicted, the neighborhood control subjects tended to learn the global-choice strategy, but the subjects with a history of heavy drug use did not.

The results support the local versus global analysis of addiction in that differences in how people performed on a laboratory procedure that pitted the local equilibrium against the global equilibrium predicted differences in drug use, particularly the likelihood that experimentation with an illicit drug would graduate into a pattern of frequent use. The results are also consistent with the prediction that cognitive differences play a role in the etiology of addiction. The control subjects had stayed in school longer (sixteen instead of thirteen years) and had higher IQs (114 and 101). The Vietnam veteran twin studies discussed earlier (Lyons et al., 2004; Toomey et al., 2003) suggest that these differences were in place prior to drug use. However, there is no way to know for sure.

The two experiments show the predicted relationships. Differences in a laboratory choice procedure that measured impulsivity predicted differences in smoking, and differences in a laboratory choice procedure that measured the capacity to learn the global equilibrium predicted drug use. In addition there was some evidence that the differences in performance in the laboratory procedures preceded drug use.

Society to the Rescue: Prudential Rules

We have identified several processes that provide protection against addiction. At the level of local choice, social interactions with nondrug users result in penalties for drug use. Survey results show that this effect is particularly pronounced when the social interactions are with a significant other, particularly a spouse. Research on social relations show that marriage varies as a function of temperament and personality (e.g., Eysenck, 1980), and research on temperament and personality reveals that these characteristics involve both individual differences in experience and in inheritance (e.g., Keller et al., 2005). Capacities that promote global choice also provide protection against addiction, and accordingly individual differences in these capacities predict individual differences in addiction. However, this account cannot be the whole story. There are large numbers of married addicts and even larger numbers of individuals who are single who nevertheless are not addicted. Similarly, in the experiments there is a good deal of overlap. Some addicts learn the global equilibrium, and some wait for the larger, later reward. Conversely, many nonaddicts fail to learn the more efficient global-choice solution and choose the sooner, smaller rewards. Indeed, the responses to the restaurant problem and other observations imply that most of the time most individuals adopt a local frame of reference when making choices, yet most do not become drug addicts.

These observations say that this discussion is incomplete. There must be some process or processes that have yet to be identified that prevent drug use from turning into drug abuse. In an interesting paper on choice, titled "Preferences or Principles," Drazen Prelec and Richard Herrnstein (1991) came to an analogous conclusion regarding choice in general. They considered how people deal with everyday choices, such as whether or not to buckle up the seat belt when going out for a drive. Their analysis points to the same mystery. People typically frame their options in terms of current values, ignoring the consequences of these choices on overall outcomes, yet they usually manage to get through life relatively unscathed. They somehow manage to make the right series of choices or a close approximation to the right choices. Although Prelec and Herrnstein did not frame the issues in quite the way it is being framed here, that is, of somehow managing to get by despite relying on specious features of reward, their paper provides a solution to the puzzle. What they say is that people do not really follow what is normally thought of as a decision process but instead adopt private rules of conduct. Individuals don't weigh either the long-term or short-term consequences of putting on a seat belt, they simply follow the rule: "safe drivers wear seat belts," or "I want my kids to wear seat belts when they are in the car, so I will always wear one." Their proposal can be generalized to cover all rules regarding appetites.

When it comes to appetites, individuals are not on their own. Cultural traditions and social institutions offer a wealth of information and proscriptions on how to eat, to drink, to sleep, to play, to find sexual pleasure, to intoxicate oneself, to socialize, and so on. Socially transmitted proscriptions set limits on when eating takes place, what is eaten, the sequence of foods, and how long a meal should last. Social custom establishes vegetables before dessert, which is healthier than the other way around, and cultural traditions even specify portion sizes and the rate of eating. Paul Rozin and his colleagues (2003) discovered that the French eat smaller portions of food than do Americans and take longer to eat them. Not surprisingly, the French have lower obesity rates than Americans. The cultural rules need not be very precise to yield a better rate of return than the local-choice perspective would. To see this, recall that Figure 6.3 shows that a property of voluntary behavior is that when choices are made on the basis of current value, the item that was most favored initially—prior to any recent choices—was overconsumed. Voluntary behavior and excess are partners. Thus, the rule "take less of what you like best," although simple, will always increase overall benefits.[3] In support of this analysis, most cultural teachings on how to manage appetites stress moderation, and moderation is most relevant for those items that are liked best.

Prudential rules take various forms. Social teachings on how to satisfy our various appetites are often quite explicit. There are specified times for eating meals and a widely shared understanding for what counts as a particular type of meal. Similarly, there are clearly stated restrictions and even legal rulings on where sex can take place and with whom. But prudential messages need not say anything explicit about consumption to be effective. Social roles, lifestyles, and even religious values set limits on appetites but do so without specifying particular times and places. Ideals that promote excellence in sports, motherhood, and even aspirations to sophistication set approximate limits on drug use. It is not sophisticated to be a sloppy drunk. Recall that Patty's concern that she not embarrass her daughters led her to stop selling cocaine, which in turn led her to stop using cocaine (Chapter 3). Similarly, many religions and philosophies frown on drug use because of the belief that it is incompatible with spiritual goals. Of course, not all social roles and values emphasize self-restraint. Dionysian cultural traditions encourage excess. But the social roles, ideals, and shared understandings that emphasize restraint are clearly dominant.

Finally, something needs to be said about what maintains prudential rules. At face value, that they persist is puzzling. Why should someone endorse and adhere to behavioral guidelines that are self-limiting? No one goes to jail for eating dessert before spinach. Similarly, no one goes to jail for getting drunk every night in the privacy of home or for having countless affairs. Yet, most people save dessert for last, go to bed sober, and are faithful. Evidence and logic suggest that two distinct mechanisms maintain prudential rules. First, prudential rules are inextricably linked with values, and values are embedded in signs of approval and disapproval that accompany social interactions. Although ephemeral, social gestures have a powerful impact on behavior. This is nicely illustrated in a recent study on altruism. One group of subjects, the "prize winners," were awarded about twenty dollars. They could, if they so wished, keep all the money for themselves or share it with an anonymous person whom they would never encounter. Half of the anonymous recipients were instructed to write a note back to the prize winners, commenting on their generosity. The prize winners were about twice as likely to share their winnings evenly when they anticipated the written feedback (Ellingsen & Johannesson, 2008). For the prize winners, the knowledge that an unknown person whom they would never meet might disapprove of their selfishness was enough to inspire generosity. Notice that the feedback operated immediately upon receipt of the gift, and that there were no long-term concrete consequences for either generosity or selfishness. The consequences were limited to the prize winner's current self-reflections. The consequences could not have been more immediate or more local. Thus, prudential rules are in part supported by socially mediated rewards and penalties that operate locally.

Second, as substitutes for global cost-benefit analyses, prudential rules offer the same advantages as the economic analyses. The results may not be as exact, but given the finding that simply restricting intake of what you like best (see Figure 6.3) pushes overall welfare toward the global equilibrium, prudential rules should generally improve overall welfare. These advantages will in turn reinforce the behaviors that produced them. Accordingly, prudential rules should prove self-reinforcing. The logic here is the same as the logic that says that voluntary behavior should reinforce abstract thought and patience. This is not to say that prudential values are always beneficial, but rather that the reward structure of voluntary behavior sets in motion processes that tend to support prudential rules that favor self-restraint.

Prudential rules, then, fill a gap. The biases inherent to local choice can lead to seriously inefficient self-destructive outcomes. Global choice solves these problems, but global choice is often unfeasible because of the large number of possible options and their abstract nature. Prudential rules offer a simple shortcut. Although it is a one-size-fits-all solution, rules that encourage self-restraint will in general push preference in the direction of the global equilibrium. Prudential rules, then, are reinforced by the benefits that come with the global equilibrium, and they are also reinforced on a moment-to-moment level by their social implications.

Individual differences in susceptibility to prudential rules. According to this discussion, we can test the role of prudential rules on drug use by evaluating the correlations between drug use and certain social roles and religious beliefs. The available data are supportive, but it needs to be pointed out that this is an area of study that has received little attention. Consequently, the studies have not yet had the opportunity to include control conditions that would support more definitive conclusions.

A number of researchers have looked at the relationships between drug use and measures of conventionality, conservatism, religiosity, and spirituality (e.g., Galaif et al., 2007; Galaif & Newcomb, 1999). Subjects filled out questionnaires that probed for information about church attendance, frequency of praying, ideas concerning the nature of God—for example, whether God punishes evildoers—and ideas about the purpose of life. Since religions often teach beliefs and practices that are incompatible with heavy drug use, the prediction is that higher levels of religiosity will be correlated with lower levels of drug use.

Researchers from the University of Virginia tested this hypothesis in a large sample, drawn from the general population (Kendler et al., 1997). The investigators were particularly interested in the relationship between answers on the religious questionnaire and situations that were likely to promote drug use, such as getting laid off from work and losing a place to live. The independent variables included frequency of church attendance, religious affiliation, frequency of private prayer, literal belief in the Bible, belief in a God that rewards and punishes, belief in the possibility of being "born again," and concern with spiritual goals.

Religiosity and drug use were negatively correlated. Those who prayed frequently and who endorsed the idea of a God who rewards and punishes reported lower levels of use or dependence on cigarettes and alcohol. The researchers' hunch that religion would play a role in times of stress was also confirmed. According to self-reports, stressful events typically increased smoking and drinking. But for those who strongly endorsed a belief in a spiritual world, there was no stress-related increase in drug use. An interesting feature of this result was a dissociation between "consciousness of a religious purpose" and religious denomination. Those who attended fundamentalist churches or believed in a God that rewards and punishes were just as vulnerable to stress-induced increases in drug use as were the nonreligious. However, those who endorsed spiritual goals were less likely to report increased levels of drug use in stressful situations. These results were later replicated in a similarly large, nonclinic community sample (Newcomb et al., 1999). In the second study, conducted in Southern California, high marks on a social conformity scale weakened the correlation between psychological distress and polydrug use. Those who more strongly endorsed the importance of obeying the law and religious commitment were less likely to turn to drugs after suffering a personal setback.

The Virginia and Southern California results are representative of the research on values and drug use. Those who express a commitment to spiritual and religious values report lower levels of drug use, particularly in stressful situations that promote excessive drug use (e.g., Gartner et al., 1991). For instance, in a review of this literature, William Miller (1998) concluded: "The correlation between spiritual/religious involvement and lower risk is one of the more consistent (although seldom taught) findings of the addiction field" (p. 982). Stanton Peele (1987) has made much the same point, noting that antidrug programs that ignore values are disarming themselves of a potentially useful tool in reducing drug use.

Among the few researchers who have looked at the relationship between values and drug use, there is no disagreement as to the empirical findings. Church attendance, spiritual values, and adherence to many traditional social roles are correlated with lower addiction rates. What this chapter adds to these observations is a hypothesis as to why spiritual values matter. The proposal is that religious values and traditional roles have a prudential component. The prudential aspects of religious values recommend consumption levels that are closer to the ideal global levels than those recommended by local bookkeeping. The gain relative to the local equilibrium reinforces the religious beliefs. The beliefs make things better and thereby persist.

These ideas are highly schematic. Religions vary markedly in terms of what they have to say about alcohol consumption and drug use, and religions do not have a monopoly on values that pertain to drug use. Some prudential rules based in religion may be so severe and simplistic that for most people they push drug consumption to levels that are less beneficial than those recommended by nonreligious, secular values. Nevertheless, the connection between religious values and drug use illustrates a point. We want to know why so many people who have access to addictive drugs do not become addicted to them, even though from a local-choice perspective, the drug is often the best choice. Religious values typically teach self-restraint and sobriety. For those who endorse religious values, this settles the issue. They do not have to weigh either the short- or long-term consequences of drug use. Rather, they have to decide whether or not they are religious or whether the religious proscriptions apply to the current situation. These turn out to be simpler decisions than whether or not to have a drink. Thus, the prediction is that differences in adherence to religious values is correlated with differences in drug use. The data support the predictions. However, it also should be added that as socially transmitted prudential rules are not tailored to individuals but set standards for populations, they will often prove a less-than-perfect solution to finding the right consumption levels.

How Rationality and Social Proscriptions
Combine to Influence Drug Use

Cost-benefit analysis involves abstract thought processes, such as keeping track of variables, considering alternatives, and tracking down contingencies. In contrast, applying prudential rules is a matter of judging similarities (Prelec & Herrnstein, 1991). Which rule best fits the case at hand? This is the job of judges and rabbis, not economists. Although different in nature, these two approaches to appetites may work together so that drug use typically reflects both types of thinking. The "sober citizen" drinks little, avoids heroin, and maybe tries marijuana a few times. The "wild and crazy guy" can't get enough of whatever drug comes his way. However, social identities are sketchy when it comes to specifics. A "sober guy" can abstain, drink once a week, have a beer each night, or perhaps even get really drunk once in a while. A moderate drinker who gets loaded once a year on New Year's Eve would still be a moderate drinker. Thus, someone who identifies him- or herself as "sober" actually has a range of drug consumption levels to choose from. At this point, the social role (prudential rule) is mute and decision making takes over. The "sober guy" sorts through the range of possible consumption levels, settling in at the one that seems best given his preferences and situation. Alternatively, it is in principle possible to review a wide range of possible consumption rates, testing many until by trial and error the ideal rate is settled on.

However, this seems unlikely because social influences are impossible to rule out, and trial and error may never locate the right level, given the complexities of choice. For example, perhaps one of the reasons people have a difficult time sticking to a diet is that they keep reviewing their options in terms of the costs and benefits rather than sticking to a rule, regardless of the apparent costs and benefits.

According to the scenario described above, drug use in general and addiction in particular are intimately linked to social values. An addict has either never subscribed to or has abandoned the values that recommend controlled drug use. Thus, despite the fact that drug use in addicts remains voluntary, it seems likely that differences in rationality, such as the ability to carry out cost-benefit analyses, do not play a dominant role in who becomes an addict. Rather, according to this theory, self-identity and values substitute for rationality.

Treatment

Although most addicts eventually quit using drugs at clinically significant levels by about age 30 and often do so without professional assistance, there is much to be gained by programs that cut short self-destructive drug use. The gains are all correlates of the fact that heavy drug use is dangerous, destructive to others, and destructive to oneself. Drug use typically starts in the late teens and early twenties, during the years that people are establishing patterns of behavior that are likely to have lifelong effects. They are in school, starting new jobs, perhaps even starting families. A regular regime of intoxication and illegal behavior is incompatible with these foundational activities, and the longer it lasts the more difficult it is to reverse its ill effects. The time lost is unrecoverable. These are not just an outsider's scoldings. That most addicts quit and virtually all make some attempt to quit means that addicts themselves typically end up regretting the time and money "wasted" on drugs. The pattern of periods of drug use and abstinence makes the same point. It also should be pointed out that the costs are not just psychological. Drug use is a vector for serious health problems, including HIV/AIDS, hepatitis, and, of course, overdoses. For those with a history of delinquency, periods of heavy drug use function as a catalyst, markedly increasing rates of criminal activity. The theme binding these concerns is that we want to live in an environment that fosters productive lives. Extended periods of heavy drug use are not productive, and they undermine productive activities that could take place during periods of sobriety, as well as the chances that others might have of pursuing more satisfying lives. As the emperor of China noted in response to the first recorded drug epidemic, "addiction drains the community of its wealth." Thus, we are obligated to do what is feasible to reduce the frequency and duration of destructive drug use.

Three types of treatment distinguish addiction from other psychiatric disorders: drug-specific pharmacological treatments, programs that arrange contingencies that devalue the drug and increase the value of nondrug alternatives, and Alcoholics Anonymous (AA) and its offshoots. The local versus global analysis helps explain why each of these approaches has something to offer and why these treatments emerged for addiction but not other psychiatric disorders.

Dole and Nyswander, who championed methadone, a pharmacological treatment for heroin addiction, proposed that they were curing a metabolic disease (e.g., Dole & Nyswander, 1967). Almost a half-century later, however, there is still no evidence that heroin addicts suffer from an opiate-related metabolic dysfunction. Rather, methadone reduces the reward value of heroin, binding to the same receptors as opiates and in so doing blunting their intoxicating effects (and also blunting withdrawal symptoms). These actions rob heroin of its capacity to function as a reward, thereby making it a less desirable choice. Nicotine replacement treatments work analogously. Disulfiram, the first pharmacological treatment for alcoholism, blocks the metabolism of alcohol so that a drink produces toxic reactions similar to those experienced by Asians who have the allele that leads to the buildup of toxic acetaldehyde. The common element in each of these treatments is that the pharmacological agents reduce the reward value of the drug. This makes perfect sense from the perspective that addiction is voluntary drug use. Devise a treatment that makes the drug less rewarding, and drug use will decrease in addicts. In contrast, pharmacotherapies for other psychiatric disorders work differently. Note that the primary symptom of addiction is drug use. Thus, if pharmacotherapies for other psychiatric disorders followed the addiction model, the goal would be to find a drug that made the symptoms less rewarding. This makes little sense. As far as we can tell, schizophrenics do not choose to have hallucinations, and those suffering from anxiety do not choose to feel uncomfortable.

The treatment programs that provide explicit advantages for abstinence and penalties for drug use are literal translations of the data presented in Chapters 4 and 5 on the correlates of quitting and the nature of addiction. If addiction is voluntary drug use, then altering the consequences of drug use will alter its frequency. Programs that have taken this approach have had considerable success. Figure 4.8 showed that when the negative consequences of drug use were insured by random testing, physicians and pilots stopped using drugs, even though prior to this contingency their drug use had been so flagrant that it came to the attention of their colleagues. The Vermont treatment program, introduced in Chapter 5, rewarded abstinence with relatively inexpensive vouchers and encouraged hobbies and social relations that offered opportunities for personal growth. As shown in Figure 5.2, cocaine addicts were willing to trade getting high for the vouchers, and the new nondrug activities squeezed out drug use. These results make perfect sense from the point of view that addicts are voluntary drug users. In contrast, for schizophrenics and OCD patients, voucher programs are not a clinical option. They are not in a position to turn in a symptom-free week for a chance to take a cooking class. It would make no sense to offer prizes for not exhibiting tics. Disease symptoms are not the sort of thing you can barter, but you can barter addiction symptoms for a voucher.

AA is a self-help group that came into prominence in the mid-twentieth century. It was started by two alcoholics in Akron, Ohio, in 1935 and has since grown into a worldwide, multimillion-member organization. Its treatment program has also become a model for other addiction self-help programs (e.g., Cocaine Anonymous). However, the organization's success is not due to corporate sponsors, government money, or any other form of outside support. Rather, it is supported by donations from members. AA reflects its members' interests, and its members are alcoholics.

In research circles AA has been notorious for not evaluating itself and for not supporting studies of its effectiveness. However, several recent studies provide evidence that AA works. The most convincing report used statistical techniques to evaluate the nature of the correlation between AA membership and sobriety (McKellar et al., 2003). The study was longitudinal and managed to recruit more than 2,000 subjects. The statistical analyses indicated that the correlation between sobriety and AA membership was a function of engaging in the AA programs. The idea that AA's success is really a function of the individual characteristics of those who choose to stay in AA (and not what they do in AA) was not supported by the data. In a review of recent studies, George Vaillant (2005), an expert on alcoholism, concluded that "Alcoholics Anonymous appears equal to or superior to conventional treatments" (p. 431).

AA's approach is multifaceted. Their nightly meetings establish a rewarding, social alternative to drinking. This is critical because for many alcoholics socializing and alcohol are joined at the hip. Alcohol lessens their social anxieties, paving the way for more spontaneous and enjoyable social interactions. The alcohol-free gatherings helped socially anxious alcoholics confront and overcome their fears. But the meetings assume that some degree of abstinence has been established, and according to the discussion of quitting in Chapter 6, the first days of abstinence are the most difficult. AA practices help the new members overcome this challenge in several ways. First, all new members have a sponsor or mentor to whom they can turn when they feel that they have to have a drink. The contact functions as an alternative or distraction, reorienting attention to something other than alcohol. Similarly, people learn to cope with discomfort or even pain by finding a distracting activity to occupy their thoughts. Second, at the meetings, new AA members meet people who had drinking problems similar to theirs but who now are sober. The meetings demonstrate that it is possible to quit and that quitting leads to a better overall existence. The old members are persuasive role models for the new members. Third, AA's emphasis on faith in higher powers can be seen as a mechanism for instilling hope. AA claims that if an alcoholic has faith, he or she can become sober. For some, the statement itself is reassuring, and for all the statement is reinforced by the successes of sober AA members. Fourth, AA offers its members opportunities for successful and meaningful social relations outside of the nightly meetings. Older members sponsor new members. They provide support, guidance, and friendship. In many instances, the relationships are productive and meaningful. My hunch is that for some AA members, sponsorship may be among their most successful human interactions and a source of pride. According to the analysis of quitting in Chapter 6, both hope and alternatives to drugs are what is needed. AA offers both.

AA programs have not emerged spontaneously for diabetes, Alzheimer's disease, heart disease, or any of the other chronic diseases that supporters of the disease interpretation say addiction is similar to. Although it is reasonable to suppose that many chronic disease sufferers would benefit from socializing with others who suffer from similar ailments, it is not reasonable to suppose that such meetings would also prove effective treatments. Clinicians do not tell individuals suffering from depression to hang out with other sufferers of depression, but they do recommend AA for alcoholics, and according to recent research with good reason.

The account of addiction presented in this book moved from empirical studies, such as the large national surveys of psychiatric health, to an analysis of the nature of voluntary behavior, and then back to empirical findings, such as spontaneous recovery, the role that dopamine plays in motivated behavior, and decreases in the prevalence of smoking. The studies presented in the earlier chapters revealed that self-destructive drug use was typically not a chronic disorder and that the correlates of quitting were the sort of factors that influence many of our decisions. In Chapter 3, addicts explained that they stopped using drugs because of concerns about income, family, and the endless hassles of scoring drugs. The findings of the large, scientific psychiatric surveys supported these statements. Addicts quit outside of the purview of clinics, which is what one would expect if the matters of everyday life are what brought drug use to a halt. Biographical, epidemiological, ethnographic, and clinical research led to the same conclusion: addicts are not compulsive drug users. They choose to keep using drugs, and they can—and do—choose to quit.

Although this account of addiction is supported by converging and complementary sources of information, it is deeply puzzling. Addiction is a form of self-destructive behavior. No one would choose to be an addict, yet people remain addicts for years. On the assumption that voluntary behavior is rational, this makes no sense. The contradiction called for a re-examination of voluntary behavior. The results revealed that voluntary action does not necessarily produce the best outcome. Voluntary action is regulated by two equilibrium states, which under certain circumstances call for conflicting choices. Addictive drugs exacerbate the conflict between the demands of the local and global equilibrium, and Figure 6.2 shows that it is possible for the best local choice to produce the worst overall outcome. Perhaps most important, the pitfalls of voluntary action are not restricted to drugs but are ever present. Whenever our choices do not conform precisely to the global equilibrium, then the deviation involves too much of the most preferred item. This helps explain the age-old problems of consumerism and excessive appetites in general. This view of voluntary behavior is supported by data as well as logic, but it is not the image of voluntary behavior that informs rational models of choice, such as those found in economics textbooks.

The analysis of voluntary behavior revealed both a dark side and a bright side to the problem of addiction. On the dark side, the conflicting claims of the local equilibrium and the global equilibrium set in motion conflicting motives that are experienced as ambivalence. On the dark side, it is possible to continue to make the best choice from a local perspective and end up at the worst possible outcome (as shown in Figure 6.2). And on the dark side, voluntary action implies that excessive consumption levels are endemic. On the bright side, voluntary behavior is an engine for change. Given the natural bias for local-choice bookkeeping, the global equilibrium establishes incentives for practices that encourage a shift to the global equilibrium. These practices include a more reflective approach to decision making, self-control, and the emergence of social traditions that encourage healthy levels of temperance. As we are almost always engaged in voluntary behavior, the pressure for positive change is continuous. This may be one of the reasons that self-destructive drug use so often ends without formal clinical interventions.

But note that voluntary behavior encourages corrective practices that are potentially at odds with one another. Conscious self-reflection leads to new, more abstract, and sensible options, but it also often leads to the rejection of social conventions. Conversely, supporters of social traditions that preach temperance are often intolerant of individuals who do not embrace the current, conventional version of temperance. Thus, the local equilibrium and global equilibrium establish conditions that encourage behavioral change, and in so doing they also reinforce processes—namely new ways of formulating options and adherence to social custom—that are potentially at odds with one another. This observation reinforces the point that voluntary actions are not only instrumental actions but are also generative actions.

Many of the addiction studies presented in this book are not well known, but are, nevertheless, well established as measured by the criterion that the results have been replicated by other researchers. Similarly, the research on the matching law (referred to in these chapters as the local equilibrium) is not well known outside of experimental psychology, yet it is one—if not the most—robust result in the study of choice. The two literatures complement one another. Research on drug use implies that individuals repeatedly make choices that are not in their long-term interests and that they themselves often regret. Laboratory and natural-setting experiments reveal that individuals make their choices on the basis of the current values of the available items. Depending on the experimental conditions, this can lead to seriously suboptimal outcomes. The results are orderly, mathematical, but not necessarily rational. In terms of their origins, the two research traditions could hardly be more different. One uses questionnaires, recruits thousands of anonymous subjects, and relies on complex, multivariate statistics. The other uses laboratory equipment and about eight subjects per experiment, and fits the results to simple mathematical models with at most two or three independent variables, but usually just one. Nevertheless the population trends and lever-pressing rates tell the same story: choice tends to produce less than optimal outcomes. Addiction is a disorder of choice.

NOTES

1. Responses to Addiction

1. Historians point out that the bill served a variety of political purposes (Courtwright, 1982; Musto, 1973) and that the bill focused on tax collection and recordkeeping with not a word about addiction or recreational drug use. However, as noted in the text, it was interpreted by the Justice Department as authorization to put a halt to nonmedical use of addictive drugs.

2. Just a few years later, across the Atlantic, the British government came to just the opposite opinion. On the recommendation of a physician-led study, the British government decided that medical doctors could prescribe heroin to heroin addicts (Musto, 1973). As suggested by the fact that two historically connected, English-speaking countries came to opposite conclusions regarding the nature of addiction, the legal rulings did not end the discussion. For the last hundred years or so there has been a steady stream of articles and books on how to classify addiction. In 2007, an Internet search on the sentence "addiction is a disease" triggered 61,700 hits, whereas the counterhypothesis, "addiction is not a disease" triggered 10,100 hits.

3. In 2008 the population of the United States exceeded 300 million. Approximately 225 million (75 percent) were 18 years old or older, and of this group, 10 percent had a history of abuse and/or dependence.

4. This figure is based on the 2001 ONDCP report and population estimates by the U.S. Census.

5. For a useful summary of the costs of substance abuse that includes alcohol as well as tobacco, see "Substance Abuse: The Nation's Number One Health Problem," prepared by the Schneider Institute for Health Policy at Brandeis University and sponsored by the Robert Wood Johnson Foundation, 2001.

6. The data were collected as part of the National Survey on Drug Use and Health (SAMHSA 1995, 2006), which is described as the major source of information on drug use in the United States. The number of informants varies from year to year, but they always number in the tens of thousands.

2. The First Drug Epidemic

1. The sources for this history include Blum, 1969; Latimer & Goldberg, 1981; Levinthal, 1988.

2. Drugs travel to their site of action by way of the circulatory system. The longer a given amount of drug remains in the circulatory system, the more dilute it becomes, all else being equal.

3. The background for the emperor's economic concerns requires an explanation. He is pointing out a cost of heavy drug use that is often overlooked. Silk, tea, and silver are goods that were resold at a profit or manufactured into products that brought profits. Opium literally as well as metaphorically went up in smoke. As the opium was exported from India to China by the British, everyone gained but the Chinese. They traded capital goods for a few hours of pleasure. Hence, from the government's perspective, opium not only sapped the faculties of its citizens, it also sapped the country of its wealth while increasing the wealth of competitors.

   The second ban against opium smoking was also ignored. In response the government attempted to prevent the British from bringing opium into China. The British complained that their rights to free trade were being infringed upon and war between the two countries broke out. The Chinese forces were greatly outmatched by British artillery. Opium continued to pour into China, and the Chinese opiate addiction problem continued to grow.

4. See, for example, the following papers: Feingold & Rounsaville, 1995; Hasin et al., 2006; Horton et al., 2000; Helzer, 1985; Helzer et al., 1987; Spitzer et al., 1980.

5. See, for example, the following papers: Anthony & Helzer, 1991; Bickel & Marsch, 2001; Kirby et al., 1999; Volkow et al., 1997; Warner et al., 1995.

6. The lifetime use data were obtained from tables published in the 2002 National Survey on Drug Use and Health (SAMHSA, 2003), and the lifetime addiction percentages were obtained from a summary of the most recent national survey on alcohol and drug dependence and their correlates (NESARC, Conway et al., 2006; Hasin et al., 2007; Stinson et al., 2005).

7. The study recruited approximately 20,000 subjects and was conducted between 1980 and 1984 (Robins & Regier, 1991).

8. In each of the studies, the biological tests were performed on a large number of women, sampled either consecutively or randomly over a set time period. For example, in a study conducted in a Detroit hospital, meconium was sampled from every other neonate born between November of 1988 and September of 1989, yielding a total of 3,010 samples (Ostrea et al., 1992).

9. Figure 2.4 summarizes the results from fourteen different studies. The studies were conducted in the locations indicated in the figure. In a few instances, dif-

ferent researchers evaluated drug use in the same city or region of the country (e.g., Land & Kushner, 1990; Ostrea et al., 1992), and in one instance, the same research group obtained metabolic measures of cocaine use in the same hospital at different times (McCalla et al., 1995). The following list identifies the study that provided the data for the locations identified in the figure, moving from the top to the bottom panel: Detroit (Ostrea et al., 1992), Baltimore (Nair et al., 1994), NYC (Matera et al., 1990), Detroit* (Land & Kushner, 1990), NYC (T1) (McCalla et al., 1995), NYC (T2) (McCalla et al., 1995), Bronx (Schulman et al., 1993), Rochester (Ryan et al., 1994), Hartford (Rosengren et al., 1993), St. Paul (Yawn et al., 1994), Hartford* (Fenton et al., 1993), Salt Lake City (Buchi et al., 1993), Urban Alabama (Pegues et al., 1994), Urban Alabama* (George et al., 1991), Rural Alabama (Pegues et al., 1994), Rural Alabama* (George et al., 1991), Rural Florida (Behnke et al., 1994).

4. Once an Addict, Always an Addict?

1. The ECA remission rates are based on Tables 4.3 and 13.8 in Anthony & Helzer (1991); and on a paper by Regier et al. (1990). The NCS remission rates are based on Table 2 in Kessler et al. (1994), and Tables 4 and 6 in Warner et al. (1995).

2. Differential mortality rates do not explain these results either. Since the data are retrospective, differential mortality is not relevant. Even if it were relevant, death rates among addicts are not high enough to explain the data.

3. An aside is in order. Lee Robins titled her summary article on her Vietnam research project: "Vietnam veterans' rapid recovery from heroin addiction: A fluke or normal expectation?" The context for the title, she explained, was that other researchers suggested that the Vietnam opiate users were not representative of U.S. opiate users. The material presented in this chapter shows that such representation is indeed important, but not in the way her critics imagined. What has been overlooked is that if Robins had conducted her study in the conventional way, if she had recruited subjects from the clinics rather than used criteria to insure a representative sample, her results would have matched U.S. results. Vietnam veterans who were in treatment typically relapsed, just as did U.S. opiate users in treatment. Similarly, her finding that most veterans neither sought treatment nor resumed opiate use matches the survey data for individuals who became heavy drug users in the United States. Thus, to answer Lee Robins's question: "rapid recovery from heroin addiction was a normal expectation."

6. Addiction and Choice

1. The top panel displays the value of a meal as a function of how frequently it was chosen. The value of a Chinese meal was set at $(10 - 9p)$ and the value of

an Italian meal was set at $(3 + 1.5p)$, where p is the proportion of choices for the Chinese meal in the last 10 meals. The bottom panel displays the value of the possible combinations of Chinese and Italian meals. The equation is $10[p(10 - 9p)] + 10[(1 - p)(3 + 1.5p)]$, where p is the proportion of Chinese meals and $(1 - p)$ is the proportion of Italian meals. The value/choice frequency relationships are the same in each panel. The only difference is in the nature of the options.

2. The problem specified that meal value varied as a function of frequency of meal choices. The graph captures this relationship by showing the frequency of Chinese and Italian meals on the horizontal axis and the value of the meals on the vertical axis. To make things more concrete, frequency was calculated over the last 10 meals. This means that each point on the horizontal axis represents n Chinese meals and $10 - n$ Italian meals. The vertical axis shows how the value of a meal changed as a function of how frequently it was chosen (according to the equations in note 1). In the top panel the vertical axis corresponds to the perspective of the person who chose which restaurant to go to on a meal-by-meal basis, which was what most people said they would do. The line sloping down from left to right is the current value of Chinese meals, and the line sloping down from right to left is the current value of Italian meals. (They slope down in opposite directions because the two types of meals are complementary.) The bottom panel shows the perspective of the few people who took into consideration that they might be better off if they selected the Chinese meal less frequently than their day-to-day preferences suggested. Hence, it shows the value of a series of Chinese and Italian meals, with the series set equal to ten for convenience. These values were obtained by combining the equations for each type of meal (see note 1). For example, the y-axis point that corresponds to two Chinese meals and eight Italian meals shows the value of a string of ten meals composed of two Chinese meals and eight Italian meals, using the values given in the top panel. Thus, the only difference between the two panels is in how the options were framed.

Each perspective led to a stable choice proportion. In the top panel this is the point at which the value lines cross. For example, to the right of the crossing point, the value of the Italian meal is higher, but choosing it makes the value of the Chinese meal higher on the next night. Correspondingly, to the left of the crossing point, the value of the Chinese meal is higher, but choosing the Chinese meal makes the value of the Italian meal higher on the next night. Thus, when someone chooses the best meal each night, choice proportions settle down to the crossing point. This is called the *local equilibrium* because it is based on current conditions. In this example, it was at 67 percent, meaning an overall preference for Chinese food. In the bottom panel the stable choice proportion is the highest point on the curve because no other choice proportion provides more meal enjoyment. This is called the *global equilibrium* because it is based on current conditions plus the impact of choice on future conditions. It was at 40 percent, meaning an overall preference in favor of Italian food. Thus, the two perspectives led to different overall choice proportions, even though the restaurants are the same and equations for value and choice frequency were the same (see note 1).

3. The equation for the value of the drug is $(14 - 0.33x)$, where x is the number of drug days. The equation for the value of nondrug competing activities is $(11 - 0.33x)$. The equation for thirty-day bundles is $30\{(p(14 - 10\,p) + [(1 - p)\,(11 - 10p)]\}$, where p is the proportion of drug days and $(1 - p)$ is the proportion of nondrug days.

4. This may not always be true. There is a character in *To Kill a Mockingbird* who is addicted to morphine and dying of cancer. She decides she wants to die drug free. This entails a painful bout of withdrawal, which she goes through aided in part by readings from one of the book's heroes, Scout. The example suggests that values play an important role in drug use, as discussed in the next chapter.

5. P. Vakili, personal communication, June 19, 2006.

6. The mathematics of local and global choice imply a few settings in which the local and global equilibrium are the same. See Heyman, 2003, for one example.

7. Voluntary Behavior: An Engine for Change

1. Alcohol, in contrast to the other addictive drugs, does not bind with a receptor, but somehow indirectly interacts with GABA receptors.

2. Of course, if both members of a couple are frequent illicit drug users, then these observations do not hold.

3. Doing more of what is immediately painful, such as exercise, is also captured by "Do less of what is most pleasing," if you consider not exercising as more pleasing than exercising.

REFERENCES

Ainslie, G. (1975). Specious reward: A behavioral theory of impulsiveness and impulse control. *Psychological Bulletin, 82,* 463–496.

———— (1992). *Picoeconomics: The strategic interaction of successive motivational states within the person.* New York: Cambridge University Press.

Ainslie, G., & Monterosso, J. (2003). Hyperbolic discounting as a factor in addiction: A critical analysis. In R. E. Vuchinich & N. Heather (Eds.), *Choice, behavioural economics and addiction* (pp. 35–69). Amsterdam: Pergamon/Elsevier Science.

Alcoholics Anonymous (1939). *Alcoholics Anonymous: The story of how many more than one hundred men have recovered from alcoholism.* New York: Works Pub. Co., 1939.

American Psychiatric Association (APA) (1994). *Diagnostic and statistical manual of mental disorders: DSM-IV* (4th ed.). Washington, DC: Author.

Anthony, J. C., & Helzer, J. E. (1991). Syndromes of drug abuse and dependence. In L. N. Robins & D. A. Regier (Eds.), *Psychiatric disorders in America: The epidemiologic catchment area study* (pp. 116–154). New York: Free Press.

Bailey, P. (1916). The heroin habit. *New Republic, 6,* 314–316.

Baumol, W. J., & Blinder, A. S. (1994). *Economics: Principles and policy* (6th ed.). Fort Worth: Dryden Press.

Baxter, L. R., Jr., Schwartz, J. M., Bergman, K. S., Szuba, M. P., Guze, B. H., Mazziotta, J. C., et al. (1992). Caudate glucose metabolic rate changes with both drug and behavior therapy for obsessive-compulsive disorder. *Archives of General Psychiatry, 49,* 681–689.

Behnke, M., Eyler, F. D., Conlon, M., Woods, N. S., & Casanova, O. Q. (1994). Multiple risk factors do not identify cocaine use in rural obstetrical patients. *Neurotoxicolology and Teratology, 16,* 479–484.

Berkson, J. (1946). Limitations of the application of fourfold table analysis to hospital data. *Biometrics Bulletin, 2,* 47–53.

Bernstein, D., Penner, L. A., Clarke-Stewart, A., & Roy, E. (2005). *Psychology* (7th ed.). Boston: Houghton Mifflin.

Berridge, V. (1990). Opium and the doctors: Disease theory and policy. In R. M.

Murray & T. H. Turner (Eds.), *Lectures on the history of psychiatry* (pp. 101–114). London: Gaskell/ Royal College of Psychiatrists.

————— (1997). Two tales of addiction; opium and nicotine. *Human Psychopharmacology, 12,* S45–S52.

Bickel, W. K., & Marsch, L. A. (2001). Toward a behavioral economic understanding of drug dependence: Delay discounting processes. *Addiction, 96,* 73–86.

Bickel, W. K., Odum, A. L., & Madden, G. J. (1999). Impulsivity and cigarette smoking: Delay discounting in current, never, and ex-smokers. *Psychopharmacology, 146,* 447–454.

Biernacki, P. (1986). *Pathways from heroin addiction: Recovery without treatment.* Philadelphia: Temple University Press.

Blum, R. H. (1969). *Society and drugs; social and cultural observations.* San Francisco: Jossey-Bass.

Bohigian, G. M., Bondurant, R., & Croughan, J. (2005). The impaired and disruptive physician: The Missouri physicians' health program—an update. *Journal of the Addictive Diseases, 24,* 13–23.

Bolla, K. I., Cadet, J., & London, E. (1998). The neuropsychiatry of chronic cocaine abuse. *Journal of Neuropsychiatry, 10,* 280–289.

Bolla, K. I., McCann, U. D., & Ricaurte, G. A. (1988). Memory impairment in abstinent MDMA ("Ecstasy") users. *Neurology, 51,* 1532–1537.

Bottlender, M., & Soyka, M. (2004). Impact of craving on alcohol relapse during, and 12 months following, outpatient treatment. *Alcohol and Alcoholism, 39,* 357–361.

Bouchard, T. J., Segal, N. L., Tellegen, A., McGue, M., Keyes, M., & Krueger, R. (2003). Evidence for the construct validity and heritability of the Wilson-Patterson Conservatism Scale: A reared-apart twins study of social attitudes. *Personality and Individual Differences, 34,* 959–969.

Brecher, E. M. (1972). *Licit and illicit drugs: The Consumers Union report on narcotics, stimulants, depressants, inhalants, hallucinogens, and marijuana—including caffeine, nicotine, and alcohol* (1st ed.). Boston: Little, Brown.

Brown, R., & Herrnstein, R. J. (1975). *Psychology.* Boston: Little, Brown.

Brownsberger, W. N. (1997). Prevalence of frequent cocaine use in urban poverty areas. *Contemporary Drug Problems, 24,* 349–371.

Buchi, K. F., Varner, M. W., & Chase, R. A. (1993). The prevalence of substance abuse among pregnant women in Utah. *Obstetrics & Gynecology, 81,* 239–242.

Burnett, D. G. (2007). *Trying Leviathan.* Princeton: Princeton University Press.

Burroughs, W. S. (1959). *Naked lunch.* New York: Grove Weidenfeld.

Carroll, K. M., & Rounsaville, B. J. (1992). Contrast of treatment-seeking and untreated cocaine abusers. *Archives of General Psychiatry, 49,* 464–471.

Carter, B. L., & Tiffany, S. T. (2001). The cue-availability paradigm: The effects of cigarette availability on cue reactivity in smokers. *Experimental and Clinical Psychopharmacology, 9,* 183–190.

Caulkins, J. P., & Reuter, P. (2006). Reorienting U.S. drug policy. *Issues in Science and Technology, 23,* 79–85.

Caulkins, J. P., & Sevigny, E. L. (2005). How many people does the U.S. imprison for drug use, and who are they? *Contemporary Drug Problems, 32,* 405–428.

Centers for Disease Control and Prevention (2006). *HIV/AIDS surveillance report 2006.* Vol. 18. Atlanta: U.S. Department of Health and Human Services. Retrieved June 28, 2008, from http://www.cdc.gov/hiv/topics/surveillance/ resources/reports.

Chasnoff, I. J., Landress, H. J., & Barrett, M. E. (1990). The prevalence of illicit-drug or alcohol use during pregnancy and discrepancies in mandatory reporting in Pinellas County, Florida. *New England Journal of Medicine, 322,* 1202–1206.

Cloninger, C. R. (1987). Neurogenetic adaptive mechanisms in alcoholism. *Science, 236,* 410–416.

Conway, K. P., Compton, W., Stinson, F. S., & Grant, B. F. (2006). Lifetime comorbidity of DSM-IV mood and anxiety disorders and specific drug use disorders: Results from the National Epidemiologic Survey on Alcohol and Related Conditions. *Journal of Clinical Psychiatry, 67,* 247–257.

Coombs, Robert H. (2007). *Drug-impaired professionals.* Cambridge, MA: Harvard University Press.

Courtwright, D. T. (1982). *Dark paradise: Opiate addiction in America before 1940.* Cambridge, MA: Harvard University Press.

Courtwright, D., Joseph, H., & Des Jarlais, D. (1989). *Addicts who survived: An oral history of narcotic use in America, 1923–1965.* Knoxville: University of Tennessee Press.

Crowley, T. (1986). Doctor's drug abuse reduced during contingency-contracting treatment. *Alcohol and Drug Research, 6,* 299–307.

D'Angio, M., Serrano, A., Rivy, J., & Scatton, B. (1987). Tail pinch stress increases extracellular DOPAC levels (as measured by in vivo voltammetry) in the rat nucleus accumbens but not frontal cortex: Antagonism by dizaepam and zolpidem. *Brain Research, 409,* 169–174.

Darke, S. (1998). Self-report among injecting drug users: A review. *Drug and Alcohol Dependence, 51,* 253–263.

Davison, M., & McCarthy, D. (1988). *The matching law: A research review.* Hillsdale, NJ: Lawrence Erlbaum Associates.

Day, H. B. (1868). *The opium habit; with suggestions as to the remedy.* Harper.

de Wit, H., & Richards, J. B. (2004). Dual determinants of drug use in humans: Reward and impulsivity. *Nebraska Symposium on Motivation, 50,* 19–55.

Dickens, C. (1974). *The Mystery of Edwin Drood.* Harmondsworth, England: Penguin Books. (Originally published 1870.)

Dole, V. P., & Nyswander, M. E. (1967). Heroin addiction—a metabolic disease. *Archives of Internal Medicine, 120*, 19–24.

Dols, M., Willems, B., van den Hout, M., & Bittoun, R. (2000). Smokers can learn to influence their urge to smoke. *Addictive Behaviors, 25*, 103–108.

Domino, K. B., Hornbein, T. F., Polissar, N. L., Renner, G., Johnson, J., Alberti, S., et al. (2005). Risk factors for relapse in health care professionals with substance use disorders. *Journal of the American Medical Association, 293*, 1453–1460.

Ellingsen, T., & Johannesson, M. (2008). Anticipated verbal feedback induces altruistic behavior. *Evolution and Human Behavior, 29*, 100–105.

Eysenck, H. J. (1980). Personality, marital satisfaction, and divorce. *Psychological Reports, 47*, 1235–1238.

Feingold, A., & Rounsaville, B. (1995). Construct validity of the dependence syndrome as measured by DSM-IV for different psychoactive substances. *Addiction, 90*, 1661–1669.

Fenton, L., Mclaren, M., Wilson, A., Anderson, D., & Curry, S. (1993). Prevalence of maternal drug use near time of delivery. *Connecticut Medicine, 57*, 655–659.

Fletcher, R. & Mayle, P. (1990). *Dangerous candy*. London: Sinclair-Stevenson.

Flynn, C., Sturges, M. S., Swarsen, R. J., & Kohn, G. M. (1993). Alcoholism and treatment in airline aviators: One company's results. *Aviation, Space, and Environmental Medicine, 64*, 314–318.

Freedman, D. X. (1991). Foreword. In L. N. Robins & D. A. Regier (Eds.), *Psychiatric disorders in America: The epidemiologic catchment area study* (pp. xiii–xiv). New York: Free Press.

Galaif, E. R., & Newcomb, M. D. (1999). Predictors of polydrug use among four ethnic groups: A 12-year longitudinal study. *Addictive Behaviors, 24*, 607–631.

Galaif, E. R., Newcomb, M. D., Vega, W. A., & Krell, R. D. (2007). Protective and risk influences of drug use among a multiethnic sample of adolescent boys. *Journal of Drug Education, 37*, 249–276.

Gallegos, K., & Norton, M. (1984). Characterization of Georgia's impaired physicians program treatment population: Data and statistics. *Journal of the Medical Association of Georgia, 73*, 755–758.

Ganley, O. H., Pendergast, W. J., Wilkerson, M. W., & Mattingly, D. E. (2005). Outcome study of substance impaired physicians and physician assistants under contract with North Carolina Physicians Health Program for the period 1995–2000. *Journal of Addictive Diseases, 24*, 1–12.

Gartner, J., Larson, D. B., & Allen, G. D. (1991). Religious commitment and mental health: A review of the empirical literature. *Journal of Psychology & Theology, 19*, 6–25.

Gazzaniga, M. S., & Heatherton, T. F. (2006). *Psychological science*. New York: Norton.

George, S. K., Price, J., Hauth, J. C., Barnette, D. M., & Preston, P. (1991). Drug abuse screening of childbearing-age women in Alabama public health clinics. *American Journal of Obstetrics & Gynecology, 165,* 924–927.

Goldstein, A. (1994). *Addiction: From biology to drug policy.* New York: W.H. Freeman.

Gordis, E. (1995). The National Institute on Alcohol Abuse and Alcoholism. *Alcohol Health & Research World, 19,* 5.

Grant, B. F., & Dawson, D. A. (2006). Introduction to the National Epidemiologic Survey on Alcohol and Related Conditions. *Alcohol Research & Health, 29,* 74–78.

Haber, J. R., Jacob, T., & Heath, A. C. (2005). Paternal alcoholism and offspring conduct disorder: Evidence for the "common genes" hypothesis. *Twin Research and Human Genetics, 8,* 120–131.

Hailman, J. P. (1969). How an instinct is learned. *Scientific American, 221,* 98–106.

Hanson, B. (1985). *Life with heroin: Voices from the inner city.* Lexington, MA: Lexington Books.

Hanson, G. R., Leshner, A. I., & Tai, B. (2002). Putting drug abuse research to use in real-life settings. *Journal of Substance Abuse Treatment, 23,* 69–70.

Hasin, D. S., Hatzenbueler, M., Smith, S., & Grant, B. F. (2005). Co-occurring DSM-IV drug abuse in DSM-IV drug dependence: Results from the National Epidemiologic Survey on Alcohol and Related Conditions. *Drug and Alcohol Dependence, 80,* 117–123.

Hasin, D. S., Samet, S., Nunes, E., Meydan, J., Matseoane, K., & Waxman, R. (2006). Diagnosis of comorbid psychiatric disorders in substance users assessed with the Psychiatric Research Interview for Substance and Mental Disorders for DSM-IV. *American Journal of Psychiatry, 163,* 689–696.

Hasin, D. S., Stinson, F. S., Ogburn, E., & Grant, B. F. (2007). Prevalence, correlates, disability, and comorbidity of DSM-IV alcohol abuse and dependence in the United States: Results from the National Epidemiologic Survey on Alcohol and Related Conditions. *Archives of General Psychiatry, 64,* 830–842.

Helzer, J. E. (1985). A comparison of clinical and diagnostic interview schedule diagnoses: Physician reexamination of lay-interviewed cases in the general population. *Archives of General Psychiatry, 42,* 657–666.

Helzer, J. E., Spitznagel, E. L., & McEvoy, L. (1987). The predictive validity of lay Diagnostic Interview Schedule diagnoses in the general population: A comparison with physician examiners. *Archives of General Psychiatry, 44,* 1069–1077.

Hendricks, M. (1988). Addiction clue: Just say dopamine. *Science News,* July 30. Retrieved Aug. 15, 2008, at http://findarticles.com/p/articles/mi_m1200/is_n5_v134/ai_6551562.

Herrnstein, R. J. (1970). On the law of effect. *Journal of the Experimental Analysis of Behavior, 13,* 243–266.

———— (1990a). Behavior, reinforcement and utility. *Psychological Science*, 1, 217–224.

———— (1990b). Rational choice theory: Necessary but not sufficient. *Journal of the American Psychologist*, 45, 356–367.

———— (1997). *The matching law: Papers in psychology and economics*. Ed. Howard Rachlin & David Laibson. Cambridge, MA: Harvard University Press.

Herrnstein, R. J., & Heyman, G. M. (1979). Is matching compatible with reinforcement maximization on concurrent variable-interval, variable-ratio? *Journal of the Experimental Analysis of Behavior*, 31, 209–223.

Herrnstein, R. J., Loewenstein, G. F., Prelec, D., & Vaughan, W. (1993). Utility maximization and melioration: Internalities in individual choice. *Journal of Behavioral Decision Making*, 6(3), 149–185

Herrnstein, R. J., & Prelec, D. (1992). A theory of addiction. In G. Loewenstein & J. Elster (Eds.), *Choice over time* (pp. 331–360). New York: Russell Sage Foundation.

Heyman, G. M. (1982). Is time allocation elicited behavior? In M. Commons, R. J. Herrnstein, & H. Rachlin (Eds.), *Quantitative analyses of behavior, vol. 2: Matching and maximizing accounts* (pp. 459–490). Cambridge, MA: Ballinger Press.

———— (1983). Optimization theory: Close but no cigar. *Behaviour Analysis Letters*, 3, 17–26.

———— (1992). Effects of methylphenidate on response rate and measures of motor performance and reinforcement efficacy. *Psychopharmacology*, 109, 145–152.

———— (1996). Resolving the contradictions of addiction. *Behavioral & Brain Sciences*, 19, 561–574.

———— (2003). Consumption dependent changes in reward value: A framework for understanding addiction. In R. E. Vuchinich & N. Heather, (Eds.), *Choice, behavioural economics and addiction* (pp. 95–127). Amsterdam: Pergamon/Elsevier Science.

Heyman, G. M., & Dunn, B. (2002). Decision biases and persistent illicit drug use: An experimental study of distributed choice and addiction. *Drug & Alcohol Dependence*, 67(2), 193–203.

Heyman, G. M., & Gibb, S. P. (2006). Delay discounting in college cigarette chippers. *Behavioural Pharmacology*, 17(8), 669–679.

Heyman, G. M., & Herrnstein, R. J. (1986). More on concurrent interval-ratio schedules: A replication and review. *Journal of the Experimental Analysis of Behavior*, 46, 331–351.

Heyman, G. M., Keung, W., & Vallee, B. L. (1996). Daidzin decreases ethanol consumption in rats. *Alcoholism: Clinical and Experimental Research*, 20, 1083–1087.

Heyman, G. M. & Luce, R. D. (1979). Operant matching is not a logical consequence of reinforcement rate maximization. *Animal Learning and Behavior, 7,* 133–140.

Heyman, G. M., & Seiden, L. S. (1985). A parametric description of amphetamine's effect on response rate: Changes in reinforcement efficacy and response topography. *Psychopharmacology, 85,* 154–161.

Heyman, G. M., & Tanz, L. (1995). How to teach a pigeon to maximize overall reinforcement rate. *Journal of the Experimental Analysis of Behavior, 64,* 277–297.

Higgins, S. T., Budney, A. J., Bickel, W. K., Badger, G. J., Foerg, F. E., & Ogden, D. (1995). Outpatient behavioral treatment for cocaine dependence: One-year outcome. *Experimental and Clinical Psychopharmacology, 3,* 205–212.

Higgins, S. T., Budney, A. J., Bickel, W. K., Foerg, F. E., Donham, R., & Badger, G. J. (1994). Incentives improve outcome in outpatient behavioral treatment of cocaine dependence. *Archives of General Psychiatry, 51,* 568–576.

Higgins, S. T., Delaney, D. D., Budney, A. J., & Bickel, W. K. (1991). A behavioral approach to achieving initial cocaine abstinence. *American Journal of Psychiatry, 148,* 1218–1224.

Higgins, S. T., Wong, C. J., Badger, G. J., Ogden, D. E., & Dantona, R. L. (2000). Contingent reinforcement increases cocaine abstinence during outpatient treatment and 1 year of follow-up. *Journal of Consulting and Clinical Psychology, 68,* 64–72.

Hillemacher, T., Bayerlein, K., Wilhelm, J., Frieling, H., Thürauf, N., Ziegenbein, M., Kornhuber, J., & Bleich, S. (2006). Nicotine dependence is associated with compulsive alcohol craving. *Addiction, 101,* 892–897.

Hoffman, J., & Froemke, S. (Eds.) (2007). *Addiction: Why can't they just stop?* New York: Rodale Press.

Horton, J., Compton, W., & Cottler, L. B. (2000). Reliability of substance use disorder diagnoses among African-Americans and Caucasians. *Drug and Alcohol Dependence, 57,* 203–209.

Houston, A. I. (1983). Optimality theory and matching. *Behaviour Analysis Letters, 3,* 1–15.

James, William (1899). Psychology and the teaching art. In *Talks to teachers on psychology—and to students on some of life's ideals.* New York: Metropolitan Books/ Henry Holt, pp. 3–14.

Johnson, R., & Connelly, J. (1981). Addicted physicians. *Journal of the American Medical Association, 245,* 253–257.

Jorquez, J. S. (1983). The retirement phase of heroin using careers. *Journal of Drug Issues, 13,* 343–365.

Jovanovski, D., Erb, S., & Zakzanis, K. (2005). Neurocognitive deficits in cocaine users: A quantitative review of the evidence. *Journal of Clinical and Experimental Neuropsychology, 27,* 189–204.

Julien, R. (2008). *A primer of drug addiction* (11th ed). New York: Worth Publishers.

Kagan, J., Reznik, J. S., & Snidman, N. (1999). Biological basis of childhood shyness. In A. Slater & D. Muir (Eds.), *The Blackwell reader in developmental psychology* (pp. 65–78). Oxford: Blackwell.

Keller, M., Coventry, W., Heath, A., & Martin, N. (2005). Widespread evidence for non-additive genetic variation in Cloninger's and Eysenck's personality dimensions using a twin plus sibling design. *Behavior Genetics, 35,* 707–721.

Kendler, K. S., Gardner, C. O., & Prescott, C. A. (1997). Religion, psychopathology, and substance use and abuse: A multimeasure, genetic-epidemiologic study. *American Journal of Psychiatry, 154,* 322–329.

Kendler, K. S., Karkowski, L. M., Neale, M. C., & Prescott, C. A. (2000). Illicit psychoactive substance use, heavy use, abuse, and dependence in a U.S. population-based sample of male twins. *Archives of General Psychiatry, 57,* 261–269.

Kessler, R. C., Berglund, P., Demler, O., Jin, R., Merikangas, K. R., & Walters, E. E. (2005a). Lifetime prevalence and age-of-onset distributions of DSM-IV disorders in the national comorbidity survey replication. *Archives of General Psychiatry, 62,* 593–602.

Kessler, R. C., Chiu, W. T., Demler, O., Merikangas, K. R., & Walters, E. E. (2005b). Prevalence, severity, and comorbidity of 12-month DSM-IV disorders in the national comorbidity survey replication. *Archives of General Psychiatry, 62,* 617–627.

Kessler, R. C., McGonagle, K. A., Zhao, S., Nelson, C. B., Hughes, M., Eshleman, S., Wittchen, H. U., & Kendler, K. S. (1994). Lifetime and 12-month prevalence of DSM-III-R psychiatric disorders in the United States. Results from the National Comorbidity Survey. *Archives of General Psychiatry, 51,* 8–19.

Khantzian, Edward J. (1997). The self-medication hypothesis of substance use disorders: A reconsideration and recent applications. *Harvard Review of Psychiatry, 4,* 231–244.

Killen, J., & Fortmann, S. (1997). Craving is associated with smoking relapse: Findings from three prospective studies. *Experimental and Clinical Pharmacology, 5,* 137–142.

Kirby, K., Petry, N., & Bickel, W. (1999). Heroin addicts discount delayed rewards at higher rates than non-drug-using controls. *Journal of Experimental Psychology: General, 128,* 78–87.

Kolb, L., & Du Mez, A. G. (1981/1924). Prevalence and trends of drug addiction in the United States and factors influencing it (*Public Health Reports, 39,* no. 21). In G. N. Grob (Ed.), *Public policy and the problem of addiction: Four studies, 1914–1924.* New York: Arno Press.

Koob, G. F., & Le Moal, M. (2006). *Neurobiology of addiction.* London: Elsevier Academic Press.

Kozlowski, L. T. & Wilkinson, D. A. (1987). Use and misuse of the concept of craving by alcohol, tobacco, and drug researchers. *British Journal of Addiction, 82,* 31–36.

Krebs, C. P., Lindquist, C. H., Koetse, W. & Lattimore, P. (2007). Assessing the long-term impact of drug court participation on recidivism with generalized estimating equations. *Drug and Alcohol Dependence, 91,* 57–68.

Kudadjie-Gyamfi, E., & Rachlin, H. (1996). Temporal patterning in choice among delayed outcomes. *Organizational Behavior and Human Decision Processes, 65,* 61–67.

Lambert, C. (2000). Deep cravings. *Harvard Magazine, 102,* 60–68.

Land, D. B., & Kushner, R. (1990). Drug abuse during pregnancy in an inner-city hospital: Prevalence and patterns. *Journal of the American Osteopathic Association, 90,* 421–426.

Latimer, D., & Goldberg, J. (1981). *Flowers in the blood: The story of opium.* New York: F. Watts.

Lee, H. (2002). *To kill a mockingbird.* London: HarperCollins. (Originally published 1960.)

Lelbach, W. K. (1975). Cirrhosis in the alcoholic and its relation to the volume of alcohol abuse. *Annals of the New York Academy of Sciences, 252(1),* 85–105.

Leshner, A. I. (1997). Addiction is a brain disease, and it matters. *Science, 278,* 45.

Levine, H. G. (1978). The discovery of addiction: Changing conceptions of habitual drunkenness in America. *Journal of Studies on Alcohol, 39(1),* 143–174.

Levinthal, C. F. (1988). *Messengers of paradise: Opiates and brain chemistry; the struggle over pain, rage, uncertainty, and addiction.* Garden City, NY: Anchor Press/Doubleday.

Lewis, D. C. (1991). Comparison of alcoholism and other medical diseases: An internist's view. *Psychiatric Annals, 21,* 256–265.

Liptak, A. (2008). 1 in 100 U.S. adults behind bars, new study says. *New York Times,* February 28, 2008. Retrieved June 28, 2008, from http://www.nytimes.com/2008/02/28/us/28cnd-prison.html?hp.

Luczak, S. E., Wall, T. L., Shea, S. H., Byun, S. M., & Carr, L. G. (2001). Binge drinking in Chinese, Korean, and white college students: Genetic and ethnic group differences. *Psychology of Addictive Behaviors: Journal of the Society of Psychologists in Addictive Behaviors, 15,* 306–309.

Lukas, S. E., & Renshaw, P. F. (1998). Cocaine effects on brain function. In S. T. Higgins & J. L. Katz (Eds.), *Cocaine abuse: Behavior, pharmacology, and clinical applications* (pp. 265–287). San Diego: Academic Press.

Lundqvist, T. (2005). Cognitive consequences of cannabis use: Comparison with abuse of stimulants and heroin with regard to attention, memory and executive functions. *Pharmacology, Biochemistry and Behavior, 81,* 319–330.

Lyons, M. J., Bar, J. L., Panizzon, M. S., Toomey, R., Eisen, S., Xian, H., & Tsuang,

M. T. (2004). Neuropsychological consequences of regular marijuana use: A twin study. *Psychological Medicine, 34,* 1239–1250.

Mack, A. H., Franklin, J. E. Jr., & Frances, R. J. (2003). Substance use disorders. In R. E. Hales & S. C. Yudofsky (Eds.), *The American psychiatric publishing textbook of clinical psychiatry* (4th ed., pp. 309–377). Washington, DC: American Psychiatric Publishing.

Maric, N., Myin-Germeys, I., Delespaul, P., de Graaf, R., Vollebergh, W., & Van Os, J. (2004). Is our concept of schizophrenia influenced by Berkson's bias? *Social Psychiatry & Psychiatric Epidemiology, 39,* 600–605.

Martin, S. P., Smith, E. O., & Byrd, L. D. (1990). Effects of dominance rank on d-amphetamine-induced increases in aggression. *Pharmacology, Biochemistry and Behavior, 37,* 493–496.

Matera, C., Warren, W. B., Moomjy, M., Fink, D. J., & Fox, H. E. (1990). Prevalence of use of cocaine and other substances in an obstetric population. *American Journal of Obstetrics & Gynecology, 163,* 797–801.

McCalla, S., Feldman, J., Webbeh, H., Ahmadi, R., & Minkoff, H. L. (1995). Changes in perinatal cocaine use in an inner-city hospital, 1988 to 1992. *American Journal of Public Health, 85,* 1695–1697.

McGue, M., Pickens, R. W., & Svikis, D. S. (1992). Sex and age effects on the inheritance of alcohol problems: A twin study. *Journal of Abnormal Psychology, 101,* 3–17.

McKellar, J., Stewart, E., & Humphreys, K. (2003). Alcoholics Anonymous involvement and positive alcohol-related outcomes: Cause, consequence, or just a correlate? *Journal of Consulting and Clinical Psychology, 71,* 302–308.

McLellan, A. T., Lewis, D. C., O'Brien, C. P., & Kleber, H. D. (2000). Drug dependence, a chronic medical illness: Implications for treatment, insurance, and outcomes evaluation. *JAMA: The Journal of the American Medical Association, 284,* 1689–1695.

McLellan, A. T., McKay, J., Forman, R., Cacciola, J., & Kemp, J. (2005). Reconsidering the evaluation of addiction treatment: From retrospective follow-up to concurrent recovery monitoring. *Addiction, 100,* 447–458.

Merlin, M. D. (1984). *On the trail of the ancient opium poppy.* Rutherford, NJ: Fairleigh Dickinson University Press.

Meyer, R. E., & Mirin, S. M. (1979). *The heroin stimulus: Implications for a theory of addiction.* New York: Plenum Publishing.

Miller, N. S., & Chappel, J. N. (1991). History of the disease concept. *Psychiatric Annals, 21,* 196–205.

Miller, W. R. (1998). Researching the spiritual dimensions of alcohol and other drug problems. *Addiction, 93,* 979–990.

Mintzer, M. Z., & Stitzer, M. L. (2002). Cognitive impairment in methadone maintenance patients. *Drug and Alcohol Dependence, 67,* 41–51.

Mischel, W., Shoda, Y., & Rodriguez, M. (1992). Delay of gratification in children. In G. Loewenstein & J. Elster (Eds.), *Choice over time* (pp. 147–164). New York: Russell Sage Foundation.

Mitchell, S. H. (1999). Measures of impulsivity in cigarette smokers and nonsmokers. *Psychopharmocology, 146,* 455–464.

Mobbs, D., Greicius, M. D., Abdel-Azim, E., Menon, V., & Reiss, A. L. (2003). Humor modulates the mesolimbic reward centers. *Neuron, 40*(5), 1041–1048.

Morgan, T. (1988). *Literary outlaw: The life and times of William S. Burroughs.* New York: Henry Holt.

Morning Edition. A father disappears, a daughter wonders. National Public Radio, at http://www.npr.org/templates/story/story.php?storyId=10606708.

Morse, R., Martin, M. A., Swenson, W. M., & Niven, R. G. (1984). Prognosis of physicians treated for alcoholism and drug dependence. *JAMA: The Journal of the American Medical Association, 251,* 743–746.

Musto, D. F. (1973). *The American disease: Origins of narcotic control.* New York: Oxford University Press.

Nair, P., Rothblum, S., & Hebel, R. (1994). Neonatal outcome in evidence of fetal exposure to opiates, cocaine, and cannabinoids. *Clinical Pediatrics, 33,* 280–285.

National Atlas. *Age 2000.* Adapted from U.S. Census Bureau, "Age: 2000," by Julie Meyer, Census 2000 Brief Series. Retrieved June 21, 2008, from http://www.nationalatlas.gov/articles/people/a_age2000.html.

National Institute on Drug Abuse (n.d.). *Addiction: It's a brain disease beyond a reasonable doubt* (PowerPoint presentation). Retrieved June 12, 2008, from http://www.nida.nih.gov/pubs/cj/CJAddiction.ppt.

——— (2008). *NIDA infofacts: Understanding drug abuse and addiction.* Retrieved June 9, 2008, from http://www.nida.nih.gov/infofacts/understand.html.

Nestler, E. J., Hope, B. T., & Widnell, K. L. (1993). Drug addiction: A model for the molecular basis of neural plasticity. *Neuron, 11,* 995–1006.

Newcomb, M. D. (1986). Cohabitation, marriage and divorce among adolescents and young adults. *Journal of Social and Personal Relationships, 3,* 473–494.

Newcomb, M. D., Vargas-Carmona, J., & Galaif, E. R. (1999). Drug problems and psychological distress among a community sample of adults: Predictors, consequences, or confound? *Journal of Community Psychology, 27,* 405–429.

O'Brien, C. P., & McLellan, A. T. (1996). Myths about the treatment of addiction. *Lancet, 347,* 237–240.

Office of National Drug Control Policy (ONDCP) (2001). What America's users spend on illegal drugs, 1988–2000. Retrieved June 9, 2008, from http://www.whitehousedrugpolicy.gov/publications/pdf/american_users_spend_2002.pdf.

——— (2004). *The economic costs of drug abuse in the United States 1992–2002.*

Washington, DC: Executive Office of the President (Publication No. 207303). Retrieved June 9, 2008, from http://www.whitehousedrugpolicy.gov/Search Results/SearchResults.asp?qu=economic+costs&x=0&y=0.

Olson, J. M., Vernon, P. A., Harris, J. A., & Jang, K. L. (2001). The heritability of attitudes: A study of twins. *Journal of Personality and Social Psychology, 80*, 845–860.

Ostrea, E. M. Jr., Brady, M., Gause, S., Raymundo, A. L., & Stevens, M. (1992). Drug screening of newborns by meconium analysis: A large-scale, prospective, epidemiologic study. *Pediatrics, 89*, 107–113.

Ott, P. J., Tarter, R. E., & Ammerman, R. T. (1999). *Sourcebook on substance abuse: Etiology, epidemiology, assessment, and treatment.* Needham Heights, MA: Allyn & Bacon.

Paris, R. T., & Canavan, D. I. (1999). Physician substance abuse impairment: Anesthesiologists vs. other specialties. *Journal of Addictive Diseases, 18*, 1–7.

Peele, S. (1987). A moral vision of addiction: How people's values determine whether they become and remain addicts. *The Journal of Drug Issues, 17*, 187–215.

Pegues, D. A., Engelgau, M. M., & Woernle, C. H. (1994). Prevalence of illicit drugs detected in the urine of women of childbearing age in Alabama public health clinics. *Public Health Reports, 109*, 530–538.

Prelec, D. & Herrnstein, R. J. (1991). Preferences or principles: alternative guidelines for choice. In R. Zeckhauser (Ed.), *Strategy and Choice* (pp. 319–340). Cambridge, MA: MIT Press.

Prendergast, M., Podus, D., Finney, J., Greenwell, L., & Roll, J. (2006). Contingency management for treatment of substance use disorders: A meta-analysis. *Addiction, 101*, 1546–1560.

Rachlin, H. (1997). Four teleological theories of addiction. *Psychonomic Bulletin & Review, 4*, 462–473.

——— (2007). In what sense are addicts irrational? *Drug and Alcohol Dependence, 90* (Suppl.), S92–S99.

Rachlin, H., & Green, L. (1972). Commitment, choice and self-control. *Journal of the Experimental Analysis of Behavior, 17*, 15–22.

Rapeli, P., Kivisaari, R., Kähkönen, S., Puuskari, V., Autti, T., & Kalska, H. (2005). Do individuals with former amphetamine dependence have cognitive deficits? *Nordic Journal of Psychiatry, 59*, 293–297.

Regier, D. A., Farmer, M. E., Rae, D. S., Locke, B. Z., Keith, S. J., Judd, L. L., et al. (1990). Comorbidity of mental disorders with alcohol and other drug abuse. Results from the epidemiologic catchment area (ECA) study. *JAMA: The Journal of the American Medical Association, 264*, 2511–2518.

Rettig, R., Torres, M., & Garrett, G. (1977). *Manny: A criminal-addict's story.* Boston: Houghton Mifflin.

Rinn, W. E. (1984). The neuropsychology of facial expression: A review of the neurological and psychological mechanisms for producing facial expressions. *Psychological Bulletin, 95,* 52–77.

Robins, L. N. (1993). Vietnam veterans' rapid recovery from heroin addiction: A fluke or normal expectation? *Addiction, 88,* 1041–1954.

Robins, L. N., Helzer, J. E., & Davis, D. H. (1975). Narcotic use in southeast Asia and afterward. An interview study of 898 Vietnam returnees. *Archives of General Psychiatry, 32,* 955–961.

Robins, L., Helzer, J. E., Hesselbrock, M., & Wish, E. (1980). Vietnam veterans three years after Vietnam: How our study changed our view of heroin. In L. Brill & C. Winick (Eds.), *The yearbook of substance use and abuse* (pp. 214–230). New York: Human Sciences Press.

Robins, L. N., & Murphy, G. E. (1967). Drug use in a normal population of young Negro men. *American Journal of Public Health and the Nation's Health, 57,* 1580–1596.

Robins, L. N., & Regier, D. A. (1991). *Psychiatric disorders in America: The epidemiologic catchment area study.* New York: Free Press.

Robinson, T. E., Gorny, G., Mitton, E., & Kolb, B. (2001). Cocaine self-administration alters the morphology of dendrites and dendritic spines in the nucleus accumbens and neocortex. *Synapse, 39,* 257–266.

Rosenberg, N. M., Marino, D., Meert, K. L., & Kauffman, R. F. (1995). Comparison of cocaine and opiate exposures between young urban and suburban children. *Archives of Pediatrics & Adolescent Medicine, 149,* 1362–1364.

Rosengren, S. S., Longobucco, D. B., Bernstein, B. A., Fishman, S., Cooke, E., Boctor, F., & Lewis, S. C. (1993). Meconium testing for cocaine metabolite: Prevalence, perceptions, and pitfalls. *American Journal of Obstetrics & Gynecology, 168,* 1449–1456.

Rossner, S. (1997). Chocolate—divine food, fattening junk or nutritious supplementation? *European Journal of Clinical Nutrition, 51,* 341–345.

Roth, P. (2007). *Exit ghost.* Boston: Houghton Mifflin.

Rounsaville, B. J., Anton, S. F., & Carroll, K. (1991). Psychiatric diagnoses of treatment-seeking cocaine abusers. *Archives of General Psychiatry, 48,* 43–51.

Rounsaville, B. J., & Kleber, H. D. (1985). Untreated opiate addicts. *Archives of General Psychiatry, 42,* 1072–1077.

Rounsaville, B. J., Weissman, M. M., & Kleber, H. (1982). Heterogeneity of psychiatric diagnosis in treated opiate addicts. *Archives of General Psychiatry, 39,* 161–166.

Rozin, P., Kabnick, K., & Pete, E. (2003). The ecology of eating: Smaller portion sizes in France than in the United States help explain the French paradox. *Psychological Science, 14,* 450–454.

Rutherford, J., McGuffin, P., & Katz, R. J. (1993). Genetic influences on eating attitudes in a normal female twin population. *Psychological Medicine, 23,* 425–436.

Ryan, R. M., Wagner, C. L., Schultz, J. M., Varley, J., DiPreta, J., Sherer, D. M., Phelps, D. L., & Kwong, T. M. (1994). Meconium analysis for improved identification of infants exposed to cocaine in utero. *Journal of Pediatrics, 125,* 435–440.

Salamone, J. D. (1994). The involvement of nucleus accumbens dopamine in appetitive and aversive motivation. *Behavioural Brain Research, 61*(2), 117–133.

Saudino, K. J. (2005). Behavioral genetics and child temperament. *Journal of Developmental & Behavioral Pediatrics, 26,* 214–223.

Schacter, D. L., Gilbert, D. T., & Wegner, D. M. (2009). *Psychology.* New York: Worth.

Schuckit, M. A. (1994). Low level of response to alcohol as a predictor of future alcoholism. *The American Journal of Psychiatry, 151,* 184–189.

Schulman, M., Morel, M., Karmen, A., & Chazotte, C. (1993). Perinatal screening for drugs of abuse: Reassessment of current practice in a high-risk area. *American Journal of Perinatology, 10,* 374–377.

Schwartz, J. M. (1998). Neuroanatomical aspects of cognitive-behavioural therapy response in obsessive-compulsive disorder. An evolving perspective on brain and behaviour. *The British Journal of Psychiatry, Supplement, 35,* 38–44.

Schwartz, J. M., Stoessel, P. W., Baxter, L. R., Martin, K. M., & Phelps, M. E. (1996). Systematic changes in cerebral glucose metabolic rate after successful behavior modification treatment of obsessive-compulsive disorder. *Archives of General Psychiatry, 53,* 109–113.

Selby, M. J., & Azrin, R. L. (1998). Neuropsychological functioning in drug abusers. *Drug and Alcohol Dependence, 50,* 39–45.

Seligman, M. E. P., Walker, E. F., & Rosenhan, D. L. (2001). *Abnormal Psychology* (4th ed.). New York: W.W. Norton.

Seligson, F. H., Krummel, D. A., & Apgar, J. L. (1994). Patterns of chocolate consumption. *American Journal of Clinical Nutrition, 60,* 1060S–1064S.

Shiffman, S., Engberg, J. B., Paty, J. A., Perz, W. G., Gnys, M., Kassel, J. D., & Hickcox, M. (1997). A day at a time: Predicting smoking lapse from daily urge. *Journal of Abnormal Psychology, 106,* 104–116.

Shiffman, S., Gwaltney, C. J., Balabanis, M. H., Liu, K. S., Paty, J. A., Kassel, J. D., Hickcox, M., & Gnys, M. (2002). Immediate antecedents of cigarette smoking: An analysis from ecological momentary assessment. *Journal of Abnormal Psychology, 111,* 531–545.

Shore, J. H. (1987). The Oregon experience with impaired physicians on probation. *JAMA: The Journal of the American Medical Association, 257,* 2931–2934.

Silberberg, A., & Williams, D. R. (1974). Choice behavior on discrete trials: A demonstration of the occurrence of a response strategy. *Journal of the Experimental Analysis of Behavior, 21,* 315–322.

Silverman, K., Higgins, S. T., Brooner, R. K., Montoya, I. D., Cone, E. J., Schuster, C. R., et al. (1996). Sustained cocaine abstinence in methadone maintenance patients through voucher-based reinforcement therapy. *Archives of General Psychiatry, 53,* 409–415.

Skinner, B. F. (1938). *The behavior of organisms: An experimental analysis.* New York: Appleton-Century.

Solowij, N., Stephens, R. S., Roffman, R. A., Babor, T., Kadden, R., Miller, M., Christiansen, K., McRee, B., & Vendetti, J. (2002). Cognitive functioning of long-term heavy cannabis users. *Journal of the American Medical Association, 287,* 1123–1131.

Spence, J. (1975). Opium smoking in Ch'ing china. In F. E. Wakeman & C. Grant (Eds.), *Conflict and control in late imperial China.* Berkeley: University of California Press.

Spitzer, R., & Fleiss, J. (1974). A reanalysis of the reliability of psychiatric diagnosis. *British Journal of Psychiatry, 125,* 341–347.

Spitzer, R., & Forman, J. (1979). DSM-III field trials: II. Initial experience with the multiaxial system. *American Journal of Psychiatry, 136,* 818–820.

Spitzer, R. L., Forman, J. B., & Nee, J. (1979). DSM-III field trials: I. Initial interrater diagnostic reliability. *American Journal of Psychiatry, 136,* 815–817.

Spitzer, R. L., Williams, J. B., & Skodol, A. E. (1980). DSM-III: The major achievements and an overview. *American Journal of Psychiatry, 137,* 151–164.

Steele, C. M., & Josephs, R. A. (1990). Alcohol myopia: Its prized and dangerous effects. *American Psychologist, 45,* 921–933.

Stellar, J. R., Kelley, A. E., & Corbett, D. (1983). Effects of peripheral and central dopamine blockade on lateral hypothalamic self-stimulation: Evidence for both reward and motor deficits. *Pharmacology, Biochemistry and Behavior, 18*(3), 433–442.

Stinson, F. S., Grant, B. F., Dawson, D., Ruan, W. J., Huang, B., & Saha, T. (2005). Comorbidity between DSM-IV alcohol and specific drug use disorders in the United States: Results from the National Epidemiologic Survey on Alcohol and Related Conditions. *Drug and Alcohol Dependence, 80,* 105–116.

Stinson, F. S., Grant, B. F., Dawson, D. A., Ruan, W. J., Huang, B., & Saha, T. (2006). Comorbidity between DSM-IV alcohol and specific drug use disorders in the United States: Results from the National Epidemiologic Survey on Alcohol and Related Conditions. *Alcohol Research & Health, 29,* 94–106.

Substance Abuse and Mental Health Services Administration (1995). *National household survey on drug abuse: Main findings 1993.* (Office of Applied Studies, DHHS Publication No. SMA 95-3020), Rockville, MD.

—— (2003). *Results from the 2002 National Survey on Drug Use and Health: Na-*

tional findings. (Office of Applied Studies, NHSDUA Series H-22, DHHS Publication No. SMA 03–3836), Rockville, MD.

———— (2006). *Results from the 2005 National Survey on Drug Use and Health: National findings.* (Office of Applied Studies, NSDUH Series H-32, DHHS Publication No. SMA 07-4293), Rockville, MD.

Tesser, A., & Crelia, R. (1994). Attitude heritability and attitude reinforcement: A test of the niche building hypothesis. *Personality and Individual Differences, 16,* 571–577.

Toomey, R., Lyons, M. J., Eisen, S. A., Xian, H., Chantarujikapong, S., Seidman, L. J., Faraone, S. V., & Tsuang, M. T. (2003). A twin study of the neuropsychological consequences of stimulant abuse. *Archives of General Psychiatry, 60,* 303–310.

Tsuang, M. T., Bar, J. L., Harley, R. M., & Lyons, M. J. (2001). The Harvard Twin Study of substance abuse: What we have learned. *Harvard Review of Psychiatry, 9,* 267–279.

Tsuang, M. T., Lyons, M. J., Meyer, J. M., Doyle, T., Eisen, S. A., Goldberg, J., True, W., Lin, N., Toomey, R., & Eaves, L. (1998). Co-occurrence of abuse of different drugs in men: The role of drug-specific and shared vulnerabilities. *Archives of General Psychiatry, 55,* 967–972.

U.S. Department of Health and Human Services (USDHHS) (2007). *The science of addiction.* NIH Pub No. 07-5605.

U.S. Surgeon General's Advisory Committee on Smoking and Health (1964). Smoking and health: Report of the Advisory Committee to the Surgeon General of the Public Health Service; Surgeon General's report on smoking and health. Washington, DC: U.S. Department of Health, Education, and Welfare, Public Health Service; Supt. of Docs., U.S. Government Printing Office.

Vaillant, G. E. (1995). *The natural history of alcoholism revisited.* Cambridge, MA: Harvard University Press.

———— (2005). Alcoholics Anonymous: Cult or cure? *Australian and New Zealand Journal of Psychiatry, 39,* 431–436.

Vaughan, W. (1981). Melioration, matching, and maximization. *Journal of the Experimental Analysis of Behavior, 36*(2), 141–149.

Volkow, N. D., Fowler, J. S., Wolf, A. P., & Schlyer, D. (1990). Effects of chronic cocaine abuse on postsynaptic dopamine receptors. *American Journal of Psychiatry, 147,* 719–724.

Volkow, N. D., & Ting-Kai, L. (2004). Science and society: Drug addiction: The neurobiology of behaviour gone awry. *Nature Reviews Neuroscience, 5,* 963–970.

Volkow, N. D., Wang, G.-J., & Fowler, J. S. (1997). Decreased striatal dopaminergic responsiveness in detoxified cocaine-dependent subjects. *Nature, 386,* 830–833.

Vuchinich, R. E., & Simpson, C. A. (1998). Hyperbolic temporal discounting in social drinkers and problem drinkers. *Experimental and Clinical Psychopharmacology, 6,* 292–305.

Waldorf, D. (1983). Natural recovery from opiate addiction: Some social-psychological processes of untreated recovery. *Journal of Drug Issues, 13,* 237–279.

Waldorf, D., Reinarman, C., & Murphy, S. (1991). *Cocaine changes: The experience of using and quitting.* Philadelphia: Temple University Press.

Wallace, D. G., Wallace, P. S., Field, E., & Whishaw, I. Q. (2006). Pharmacological manipulations of food protection behavior in rats: Evidence for dopaminergic contributions to time perception during a natural behavior. *Brain Research, 1112,* 213–221.

Waller, N. G., Kojetin, B. A., Bouchard, T. J. Jr., Lykken, D. T., & Tellegen, A. (1990). Genetics and environmental influences on religious interests, attitudes, and values: A study of twins reared apart and together. *Psychological Science, 1,* 138–142.

Warner, J. (1994). 'Resolv'd to drink no more': Addiction as a preindustrial construct. *Journal of Studies on Alcohol, 55,* 685–691.

Warner, L. A., Kessler, R. C., Hughes, M., Anthony, J. C., & Nelson, C. B. (1995). Prevalence and correlates of drug use and dependence in the United States. Results from the National Comorbidity Survey. *Archives of General Psychiatry, 52,* 219–229.

Weatherby, N., Needle, R., Cesari, H., et al. (1994). Validity of self-reported drug use among injection drug users and crack cocaine users recruited through street outreach. *Evaluation and Program Planning, 17,* 347–355.

Weich, S., Twigg, L., & Lewis, G. (2006). Rural/non-rural differences in rates of common mental disorders in Britain: Prospective multilevel cohort study. *British Journal of Psychiatry, 188,* 51–57.

Wilde, O., & Mighall, R. (2003). *The Picture of Dorian Gray.* Harmondsworth, England: Penguin. (Originally published 1890.)

Williams, B. A. (1988). Reinforcement, choice, and response strength. In S. S. Stevens & R. C. Atkinson (Eds.), *Stevens' handbook of experimental psychology: Learning and cognition* (2nd ed., pp. 167–244). New York: Wiley.

Yawn, B. P., Thompson, L. R., Lupo, V. R., Googins, M. K., & Yawn, R. A. (1994). Prenatal drug use in Minneapolis–St. Paul. *Archives of Family Medicine, 3,* 520–527.

Zinberg, N. E., Harding, W. M., & Winkeller, M. (1977). A study of social regulatory mechanisms in controlled illicit drug users. *Journal of Drug Issues, 7,* 117–133.

INDEX